YOUR BREASTS

YOUR BREASTS
A Complete Guide

JEROME F. LEVY, M.D.

with

DIANA ODELL POTTER

THE NOONDAY PRESS
Farrar, Straus & Giroux
NEW YORK

Copyright © 1990 by Jerome F. Levy
All rights reserved
Published simultaneously in Canada by HarperCollins*CanadaLtd*
Printed in the United States of America

First edition, 1990

Library of Congress Cataloging-in-Publication Data
Levy, Jerome F.
Your breasts : a complete guide / Jerome F. Levy with Diana
Odell Potter.—1st ed.
p.   cm.
1. Breasts—Diseases—Popular works.   2. Breast feeding.
3. Mammaplasty—Popular works.   I. Potter, Diana Odell.
II. Title.
RG492.L48   1990   618.1'9—dc20   89-77967   CIP

Chapter 5 originally appeared in slightly
different form in *Self*

To my mother and father

Contents

YOUR BREASTS

1

Introduction

A woman perceives her breasts as much more than a physical part of her body: for women as well as men, they are the embodiment of femininity and the focus of deeply felt emotions. Intense emotions are also connected with breast-feeding an infant. But for many women this experience is short-lived or may never occur, whereas the contributions of a woman's breasts to her appearance, her self-esteem, and her sexual satisfaction continue throughout her life. Small wonder, then, that when a breast problem arises, anxiety about it may inhibit a woman's ability to receive information and make decisions.

As a physician/surgeon in private practice who has specialized in breast surgery, I have seen thousands of patients with a variety of breast problems since 1963—hundreds every year—and treated hundreds of women for cancer of the breast. I have greatly admired their strength and courage, and have learned from them two lessons essential to every practitioner: the preciousness of life and the urgent need for compassion.

Most breast problems are not life-threatening and respond readily to treatment. But the current risk of developing breast cancer, among North American women, is one in ten. So, although the following chapters will cover *every* aspect of breast care, from basic anatomy to cosmetic surgery, they will also explain the techniques of self-examination, regular medical screening, and mammography for breast problems, including cancer.

Early detection and prompt treatment, if performed properly, are the most effective tools that can be used against cancer. They are the tools that will be responsible for successfully treating *90 percent of the women who will develop the disease.*

Throughout the book, illustrations and charts have been used to clarify the text wherever possible; the results of scientific studies have been included where they are relevant. I have also cited case histories. Of course, the names of patients have been changed to protect their privacy.

As my patients have helped me to become a more understanding and caring physician, I hope to help them, and every woman who reads this book, in return. First, by approaching a difficult subject with objectivity and sympathy, so that myth can be replaced by the knowledge necessary for proper breast care. And second, by supporting every woman's right to full participation in all decisions relating to her medical problems and treatment. It's amazing how often, when I see a patient as a second opinion, she will tell me her doctor never listened to her. When I see any woman for a breast problem, I try to discover what *she* perceives as being wrong. I try to respond compassionately to *all* the concerns she shares with me. It has been my experience that one of the best foundations for trust in the physician-patient relationship is dialogue; I believe that every patient has the right to take part in one.

† A WOMAN'S RIGHT TO † COMPASSIONATE CARE

Most doctors today, I believe, will make an effort to help a woman relax and discuss her breast problem fully. But, unfortunately, this positive approach still is not universal.

It is a sad fact that doctors have traditionally tended to overlook the importance of a woman's breasts, and their treatment of breast problems has sometimes been insensitive, to say the least. From the Victorian era until the social and sexual revolutions of recent times, most doctors simply told women how their breast problems would be treated—and I mean literally *told* them, with little or no concern for the woman's feelings and without involving her in the decisions. (I witnessed many such instances during my own medical school education and surgical training in the 1950s and 1960s.)

Unfortunately, women still run the risk of encountering this attitude in doctors. When women with breast problems come to me for second opinions, I sometimes hear disturbing accounts of what other doctors have told them. For example:

• "When I told my physician that I have severe pain in my breasts every month before my period, he just brushed my concerns aside and said it will get better when I reach menopause—but I'm only twenty-nine!"

- "When I told my family doctor that I wanted to consider having my breasts made larger, he laughed and told me I was stupid for wanting to change my appearance. He asked whom I was trying to impress."
- "I have a breast lump, and my doctor wants to remove it. He says if it's cancerous, he will not even discuss saving the breast and will do a mastectomy while I am still asleep. He asked me, 'Why would anyone want to go to all the trouble of having irradiation treatments just to save the breast?' "
- "I understand the need for the mastectomy (and not breast conservation) to treat the sizable cancer in my breast, but I'm also interested in breast reconstruction. My doctor asked me why I was interested in that at my age. I'm only sixty-one. Is that too old to care how I look and feel?"

The insensitivity of comments like these speaks for itself. But they can have an even more damaging effect if the woman doesn't question their "rightness" in connection with her medical problem and treatment. She should—indeed, she must—make sure she receives from her doctor *all* the information pertinent to her condition and its treatment. *Nothing in the doctor-patient relationship gives the doctor the right to dictate to a woman what she should or shouldn't think about her body or what treatment she should receive.*

I urge any woman concerned about any aspect of her medical care to press her doctor for the answers to her questions. If she does not feel completely satisfied with the answers she receives, I believe she should trust her own judgment and get a second or even a third doctor's opinion before making critical decisions concerning her diagnosis and treatment.

Mrs. Virginia Nelson, age 38, was referred to me after her first visit to a gynecologist at our hospital. She told me that about a year before, while doing a self-examination of her breasts, she felt a firmness beneath her right nipple. It just "didn't feel right," she said—it was hard and felt "like a board" compared to the softness of the same area on her other breast. It also seemed to her that the right nipple was "being pulled inside."

She immediately went to see her own gynecologist, who, after examining her, told her he'd found no problems with her breasts. Still feeling uneasy, she asked him why the right nipple looked funny. It was "mastitis," he explained; if she would just manipulate the nipple, it would come back out.

Then she asked if it might not be a good idea for her to have a mammogram, and he scheduled her for one, with apparent reluctance. "He seemed offended, as if I was questioning his judgment," Mrs. Nelson told me. "So when I came back to his office with the mammogram films and he told me the whitish area I saw behind the nipple was nothing to worry about, I decided not to 'bother' him anymore."

Six months later, Mrs. Nelson again questioned her gynecologist about the hardness and inversion of her right nipple; both seemed to have increased. Again, he told her there was "nothing to worry about." Finally, after another six months had passed, she sought the opinion of a second gynecologist, my colleague at our hospital. He immediately suspected she had a breast cancer.

Unfortunately, his suspicions were correct. Mrs. Nelson required a modified radical mastectomy, with immediate breast reconstruction. In addition, she received extensive chemotherapy. Seven of her lymph nodes contained cancer, which meant she would have an increased risk of recurring cancer. If she had sought a second opinion at the time of her initial uneasiness about her doctor's advice, she almost certainly would have had a better prognosis. Happily, since her mastectomy, she has continued to be well, but I am concerned about the future.

Mrs. Nelson had done many things "right"—practiced regular breast self-examination, reported an abnormal finding to her doctor, requested and received a mammogram, followed her doctor's advice. But she lacked the confidence to follow her own instinctive judgment, which told her something *wasn't* quite "right" with her doctor's advice. She should have sought a second doctor's opinion immediately.

Let us start at the beginning with some basic anatomy, an explanation of the stages in breast development, and what's considered "normal."

† Basic Anatomy and Function †

Each breast contains from fifteen to twenty lobules. Each lobule has milk-producing glands and a network of ever-larger ducts to collect the milk from the glands. All of the large ducts then pass through the nipple. These glands, ducts, and lobules are supported in a "fabric" of fibrous and fatty tissue that gives breasts their size and shape.

The areola (the darker area surrounding the nipple) is usu-

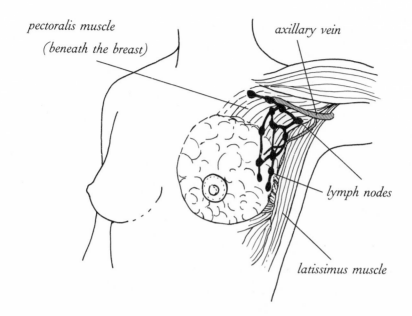

pectoralis muscle
(beneath the breast)

axillary vein

lymph nodes

latissimus muscle

DIAGRAM 1-1   Anatomy of the Breast

ally lighter in color than the nipple, but darker than the sur-rounding skin. The tiny bumps on the surface of the areola are glands. The nipple contains muscle tissue that allows it to become erect when stimulated by infant sucking, cold weather, irritating clothing, or sexual arousal. Most nipples are partially erect most of the time, but flat or even inverted nipples are also normal if they have always been that way. But if the appearance of the nipple changes, it should always be checked by a doctor.

The blood and lymph fluid in the tissues of the breast drain into small blood vessels and lymph channels. The lymph fluid then drains into the very important groups of lymph nodes located in the axilla (armpit) and beneath the breast bone, while the blood flows through veins in the armpit back to the heart and lungs, and throughout the body. (Diagram 1-1.)

† THE LIFELONG CYCLE OF †
BREAST GROWTH AND CHANGE

In infants and preschool girls, one or both breasts may temporarily enlarge due to normal changes in the hormonal balance in the child. Before puberty, a young girl's future breasts are only two small lumps, about the size of peas, located just under her nipples. From these small lumps, all the tissues of her breasts will develop. *They must never be removed in the mistaken belief that they are abnormal growths.* Before puberty, breast problems are virtually nonexistent.

† AT PUBERTY, THE ONSET †
OF BREAST DEVELOPMENT

During puberty, the glands and ducts in the breasts develop and grow in response to stimulation and regulation by the female hormones, estrogen and progesterone. These hormones, which are also responsible for the cyclical nature of menstruation, will continue to influence the breast through the woman's reproductive years and beyond. Once the glands and ducts are fully developed, the basic structure of the woman's breasts remains the same throughout her life.

During the early, "budding" stage of breast development, the young girl's breasts are typically small, pointed, and firm. Later, during adolescence and early adulthood, they become larger, softer, and more rounded. (Diagram 1-2.)

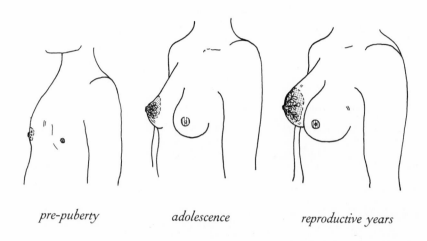

pre-puberty   *adolescence*   *reproductive years*

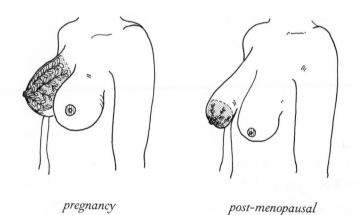

pregnancy   *post-menopausal*

DIAGRAM 1-2   The Lifelong Cycle of Breast Growth
and Change

† BREAST CHANGES DURING MENSTRUATION †

During the last two weeks of a woman's menstrual cycle, the breasts typically enlarge slightly because of fluid retention; the resulting feeling of fullness or heaviness can be painful because the ducts and glands are stretched by the fluid. With the onset of menstruation, the excess fluid is absorbed back into body tissues and the breasts return to normal size. These changes can be quite marked in some women, but in most they are relatively minor.

† THE BREASTS IN PREGNANCY AND LACTATION †

Pregnancy and lactation (the period of milk production and nursing) is the only time when a woman's breasts actually change in adulthood and function as mammary glands, so you might think that that is when problems are most likely to arise. Yet the opposite is true. Very few breast abnormalities occur during pregnancy, and only rarely does a pregnant woman or nursing mother need to consult a doctor about her breasts.

Of course, the breasts *do* change at this time, beginning early in pregnancy with a feeling of fullness and enlargement, a darkening of skin color (especially of the areolae and nipples), and the more noticeable prominence of the small glands on the surface of the areolae. The pregnant woman may have some soreness or discomfort similar to, but subtly different from, the sensations she experiences before her menstrual period begins. For maximum comfort—particularly when she exercises—she may need a support bra, in a larger-than-usual size.

Fibrocystic changes and suspicious lumps can occasionally arise in a woman's breasts during pregnancy, but they are uncommon, in part because most pregnant women are young and have not yet reached the age when breast problems most often develop. (With the trend toward having children later in life, however, more women may experience breast problems during pregnancy.)

Pregnancy does *not* cause breast cancers. The few that are discovered during pregnancy began growing several years earlier (see Chapter 8). But breast cancers that *have* been developing may become evident during pregnancy, either because they coincidentally became large enough to be detected or because their growth was stimulated by estrogen and progesterone.

During pregnancy, the body's output of estrogen and progesterone increases to very high levels, stimulating the glands in the woman's breasts to full readiness for milk production. As the baby's birth approaches, the breasts become firm—sometimes painfully hard—and lumpy; this usually ends abruptly when milk production begins. Milk is not produced until after the baby is born, although the nipples may normally discharge a clear milky fluid during the late stages of pregnancy.

As soon as the baby is born, the estrogen and progesterone levels drop precipitously, signaling the breast glands to begin milk production. The lumpiness that results when the glands fill with milk is entirely normal. When a particular lump does not subside once the milk is sucked from the breast, most often it is merely a gland or duct that has failed to empty, and simple massage may alleviate the condition. If the lump doesn't disappear, however, the doctor may aspirate the area, withdrawing the milk through a needle. If the lump does not contain milk, he may recommend a biopsy. The biopsy should not interfere with continued nursing so long as no cancer is found.

Breast care for a nursing mother is mainly a matter of washing the breasts before and after nursing to avoid exposing the infant to infection. The breasts should not be *scrubbed*, however. This can rub off the natural protective oils on the skin, drying it out and causing cracks to form that can harbor infectious bacteria.

One such organism is *staphylococcus*, the bacterium that causes the most common medical problem among nursing mothers: mastitis. This is a true infection of the nipple, breast, or both that can begin with just a small scratch or irritation of the skin or nipple. Mastitis must be treated with antibiotics, or if an abscess (a collection of pus under the skin) occurs, it must be surgically opened and drained. Properly treated, mastitis usually subsides within forty-eight hours, and nursing can be resumed at this time or soon thereafter.

† CHANGES IN THE BREASTS †
AS A WOMAN MATURES

After each pregnancy and/or as a woman grows older, the skin and tissues of her breasts tend to lose some of their elasticity, especially if her breasts are large and heavy. As a result, the breasts normally "settle" somewhat to a position lower on the chest wall (Diagram 1-1).

During and after menopause, a woman's body produces smaller amounts of estrogen and progesterone, causing cessation of her menstrual cycle and of her breasts' milk-producing capability. The breast glands and ducts shrink; there is less fluid retention and feeling of fullness in the breasts. More fat is deposited around the glands, so the breasts feel smoother.

With this reduction in hormonal breast stimulation you might expect a reduced likelihood of developing breast problems. Unfortunately, one group of problems is replaced by another. The aggravating benign problems occur less frequently, whereas breast cancer becomes more prevalent.

† What's Normal †

Sometimes a woman will ask me whether her breasts are "normal," because they seem unusually small or large to her, or because they are not exactly identical—one may be a little bigger than the other, or a little higher on the chest; the nipples may be inverted, or the nipples and areolae may not be identical in appearance. There is a simple answer to this question: *Every woman's breasts are different from every other woman's breasts, and the differences are usually "normal" as long as no medical breast problems exist.*

In addition, both lumpy and smooth breasts are normal. The breast glands and fibrous tissue can be easily felt in breasts

that are small and contain little fatty tissue; these breasts usually feel somewhat lumpy. In contrast, in large breasts with
considerable fatty tissue, the glands and fibrous tissue lie
deeper and are more hidden, so the breasts feel smooth. Also,
if a woman gains a significant amount of weight, it is normal
for some of the new fatty tissue to enlarge her breasts. The
opposite will occur if she loses weight.

What causes one woman's breasts to develop generously
and another woman's breasts to remain small? This probably
depends mainly on genetic factors, which can vary widely
even among women in the same family. Sometimes a large-
breasted woman will have a daughter with small breasts and
a granddaughter with larger ones. Normal breasts range in
weight from a few ounces each to several pounds, with most
weighing between one-half pound and two pounds.

Occasionally, during a visit to my office, a woman will
mention that she doesn't consider her breasts to be attractive
because they don't look like the breasts of the young women
in magazine advertisements and television commercials.

This concern about what's "normal" may also stem from
the fact that most women's breasts, except for differences in
size, look about the same—uplifted and firm—when clothed.
Because this is usually due to the support a bra and well-cut
clothes give the breasts, a woman may feel concern when she
is undressed and her breasts don't look like this "ideal." I can
assure you that in the course of examining many women's
breasts over a number of years, I have seen very few that

were shaped like the media would have us believe is the norm.

For almost all women, the breasts are the focus of initial sexual arousal. A woman's nipples and areolae are extremely sensitive to touch, much more so than the rest of the skin of the breasts; caressing the nipple area stimulates general sexual excitement affecting the woman's entire body.

There are many variations of "normal" responses to breast stimulation. For some women, breast stimulation is of paramount importance at the beginning of lovemaking, and they can reach great heights of arousal through their partner's initial caresses. But not all women respond this way; in fact, for some women, breast stimulation is inconsequential, and for a few, it can even be painful, especially just before the onset of menstruation, when the breasts may be sore to the touch. (This can also be a problem for a woman with fibrocystic changes in her breasts.) Each woman and her partner must work out the pattern of breast stimulation that leads to the greatest sexual satisfaction for both of them.

† TALKING WITH THE DOCTOR †
ABOUT A BREAST PROBLEM

Before I see a new patient, I review as much information as I have about her and her reason for coming to see me. When scheduling such an appointment, we always try to obtain the actual mammogram if she has had one taken. When I meet her in the examining room, I ask her to describe her problem in her own words.

A typical patient might say, "I had a mammogram because a close friend who has breast cancer insisted that I have one. My doctor informed me something abnormal had shown up in my right breast. He recommended that I see a specialist." After she tells me everything that seems relevant, I explain that the next step is for me to examine her breasts. For any woman concerned about a problem with her breasts, the doctor's physical examination is stressful. So I always take time to explain what I'm doing and answer her questions.

How much I can learn from a physical examination of a woman's breasts depends in part on their size and smoothness. The smaller, less fatty, and therefore lumpier breasts can be more difficult to examine than large, smooth breasts, because the natural lumpiness makes abnormal lumps more difficult to distinguish.

Immediately following the examination, I give the patient my overall impression of her condition and explain what I think the next step should be. At this point, I offer to show her her mammogram. If it turns out that a biopsy is required, I tell her what this procedure is and how it is performed (see Chapter 4).

While this is a very general scenario, an understanding of the basic information covered in this and the following chapters can help you take *active* care of your breasts. Remember: early detection of breast problems is the key to successful treatment and—regardless of how diagnostic and treatment methods may change—it always will be.

2

Your Guide to Breast Screening

Like most women, you probably see your family physician and/or gynecologist at least once a year for a routine checkup. You want to be *sure* you're healthy, but if a problem is developing, you want it to be caught early and resolved quickly. That's the principle behind regular screening (examination and evaluation) for breast problems, too. *I recommend that every woman have her breasts examined once or twice yearly (depending on her age) by her doctor, have mammograms at the intervals he or she recommends, and examine her own breasts monthly.* In most checkups, no problem will be found. When a problem is developing, however, regular screening almost always detects it at an early, highly treatable stage—sometimes years ahead of the time when it would otherwise become apparent.

If the problem is breast cancer, early detection can be life-saving. A number of clinical studies in the United States and Europe have proven that deaths from breast cancer decreased by 25 to 30 percent in women who underwent screening.[1] I tell my patients to think of regular breast screening as a "safety net," warding off the risk that breast cancer will progress, undetected, until it reaches a stage when treatment may not be fully successful.

† WHAT BREAST SCREENING MAY REVEAL †

A breast cancer typically has been growing for several years before it can be seen on a mammogram and even longer before it can be felt beneath the skin. So when I say "early detection," I'm referring to the "earliest possible" detection. There is no doubt that the smallest cancers are the most successfully treated, and in most cases mammography can detect a very small cancer at the earliest stage possible. (Diagram 2-1.)

Your doctor can help you plan your own breast-screening program in accordance with your age, risk factors, and other individual characteristics. After the age of 20, every woman should have a yearly professional breast examination. When you reach 30 or 35, you should have one twice a year. But this leaves too much time between examinations for breast problems to develop undetected. That's why you also need monthly self-examination of your breasts, using a systematic method (see page 27), plus mammography as recommended in Chapter 3.

† SCREENING AND DIAGNOSIS: †
WHAT'S THE DIFFERENCE?

Most often, in most women, screening doesn't diagnose; it simply (but importantly) signals that an abnormal area of breast tissue exists. To obtain the diagnosis, a needle aspiration or a biopsy must usually be performed. The needle aspiration will resolve the problem if a cyst is present; if not, the biopsy

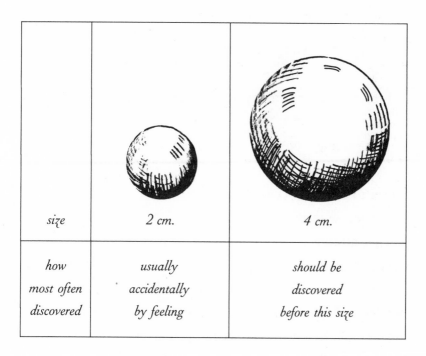

size	¹/₂ cm.	1 cm.
how most often discovered	mammography	mammography but also by careful examination

size	2 cm.	4 cm.
how most often discovered	usually accidentally by feeling	should be discovered before this size

DIAGRAM 2-1   Sizes of Breast Lumps

will remove the abnormal tissue, which can then be examined under the microscope for specific diagnostic changes in cell structure.

I wish there were a way to minimize the anxiety every woman feels when her doctor recommends a breast biopsy. Fortunately, the waiting period from discovery to biopsy to diagnosis is short, seldom more than a few days. Eighty percent of the time, biopsy turns up either a fibrocystic or other benign condition. If the diagnosis is cancer and breast screening has detected it at an early stage, I can usually give the woman an excellent outlook for successful treatment.

† The Phenomenon of Denial †

Unfortunately, despite the clear-cut value of early detection of breast problems, many women don't have regular breast screening. Some just "don't have the time." Others don't think it makes a big difference when their problem is found. But many are simply too frightened of the possibility of breast cancer to even associate themselves with it through testing or discussion with the doctor.

This attitude of "if I don't acknowledge breast cancer's existence, it won't happen to me" has no basis in fact. Ten out of 100 women will eventually get breast cancer whether they've had regular breast screening or not. And those whose cancer is discovered by chance rather than by carefully planned screening will typically have larger cancers and reduced chances of successful treatment.

Don't let this happen to you.

† Breast Screening Is Safe †

No health hazard is associated with physical examination of the breasts. In the early days of mammography, the procedure acquired a reputation for being dangerous and for increasing the risk of breast cancer because it involved much higher amounts of radiation than are used today. The very small amount of radiation used for mammography now poses absolutely no hazard and *does not* increase a woman's risk of developing breast cancer.

At present, mammography is our most effective tool for detecting breast cancer in its early, highly treatable stages. Other methods are being tested (see page 52), but none yet equals mammography's effectiveness or safety.

† What About Cost? †

Examining your own breasts costs nothing. As for the doctor's examination and mammography, the total cost is typically covered wholly or in part by medical insurance. Medicare has now begun paying for screening mammography.

Set against the risk (and ultimate high cost) of not detecting breast cancer while it's still at an early stage, this seems a small amount to pay for regular breast screening. But not all my patients can afford that amount or have insurance that will cover it, and many other women have difficulty finding the money in the family budget. Fortunately, there are alternatives to having an examination and mammogram at your doctor's office or in the hospital.

Communities periodically arrange for mobile-clinic vans to

travel to companies, shopping malls, parks, and other public places. Women can have mammograms done in a mobile clinic, usually at low cost, sometimes for as little as $25. If you're concerned about the cost of regular breast examinations, ask your doctor what community resources are available to you. Above all, never let cost keep you from seeing your doctor regularly and having mammograms at the intervals she suggests.

Finally, I suggest that you consult your doctor whenever you feel concerned about the health of your breasts, no matter when she last examined you. She won't mind a quick phone call—I never do. And she'll be glad to know that you're alert to potential problems.

† BREAST SELF-EXAMINATION: †
HOW TO DO IT AND WHY

Breast self-examination can't substitute for regular screening by your doctor and by mammography. But neither can those techniques substitute for frequent self-examination— your personal contribution to safeguarding the health of your breasts.

Breast self-examination is done monthly, just after a woman's menstrual period ends and breast swelling subsides. This chapter explains how to use the techniques of inspection and palpation (finger pressure) to examine your breasts and become familiar with their normal appearance and feel. That way you'll notice even small changes; you'll know what such a change may mean and whether or not you should make an appointment with your doctor.

† Understanding the Benefit of †
Regular Breast Self-Examination

If a lump becomes discoverable shortly after you are examined by your doctor, it may be six to twelve months before you see him again for a regular checkup. A woman who is trained in breast self-examination can usually feel almost as small a lump as her doctor.

Only about 15 percent of women who should have regular mammograms and doctor's examinations do so. As a result, accidental discovery of a breast lump by a woman while bathing or dressing is still too common. A lump noticed in this random way is typically larger than those found by monthly self-examination. If it turns out to be a cancer, its size may indicate more advanced disease.

In most but not all cases, mammography can discover a lump earlier than it can be felt. However, several times each year I feel a lump that was not seen on mammography, proving that palpation of the breasts is still very important.

† Your Guide to Correct Self-Examination †
of Your Breasts

You are the world's most knowledgeable authority on *you*—your state of mind, your capabilities, your body. So much of the time, *you're* the expert when it comes to deciding what is or is not normal for your body.

Doctors call patients' normal findings *baseline data* and value them as a basis for comparison when changes from normal occur. This concept is valuable for breast self-examination as well: by examining your breasts regularly, you become thoroughly familiar with their normal contour and "feel." Every woman's breasts are unique in their size, shape, nipple area, contour, and tissue softness. If any noticeable change from the baseline does occur, you're primed to notice it the next time you examine your breasts. If the "next time" is eleven months in advance of your next scheduled mammogram or doctor's examination, that's eleven critical months the lump doesn't have for growing and possibly spreading before it's discovered.

In a large study from a number of hospitals in Georgia, the percentage of women who survived breast cancer for five years was substantially greater for women who practiced breast self-examination (77 to 61 percent).[2]

† When's the Best Time to † Examine Your Breasts?

Your breasts feel different at different times of the month: as your menstrual period comes on, causing your breasts to swell, they feel firmer, and then after your period, they shrink back to their normal size and feel softer. The point when they're at the "lowest ebb" in this cycle—when breast glands and ducts are least stimulated by the female hormones estrogen and progesterone and therefore least prominent—is the ideal time to perform breast self-examination, every month. This is usually about a week after your period begins. (It's also the best time in the month to schedule an examination by your doctor.)

Ideally, a woman should begin monthly breast self-examination at around age 20, when she begins having regular gynecological examinations. In a woman so young, the breasts have little fat and normally feel firm and somewhat lumpy, so changes can be difficult to detect. But again, knowing what feels normal, even in lumpy breasts, is the key to detecting abnormalities.

If you're no longer menstruating but your breasts become tender at certain times of the month, pick a time in the month when they aren't tender and examine your breasts monthly on that date. If your breasts don't change at all during the month, pick an easy-to-remember date to examine them, such as the first of the month.

Finally, keep in mind that the breasts undergo changes not only during the menstrual cycle but also during pregnancy, aging, weight changes, and use of birth-control pills. A breast biopsy also alters breast contour slightly. If you have questions about how any of these conditions might affect the results of your breast self-examination, ask your doctor.

† How to Examine Your Breasts †

Along with choosing a regularly scheduled time for examining your breasts, you need to follow a regular examination technique.

If, after reading this chapter, you want to learn more about breast self-examination, I recommend attending a breast-screening clinic. These are held at local hospitals or doctors' offices or in mobile vans set up during community health drives. You should see a videotape that describes the technique, and trained instructors may demonstrate it on soft plastic models and on you. Usually the entire demonstration takes less than an hour. Your technique of breast self-examination should be very similar to your doctor's.

For a complete examination: *inspect* your breasts using a mirror and then *palpate* (feel) them—first while standing or sitting, then while lying down.

† INSPECTION †

Stand in front of a mirror, naked to the waist with your arms at your side. Look at each breast separately, then compare them. No woman's breasts are identical: one is usually larger and somewhat differently shaped than the other (Diagram 2-2).

Next, raise your arms above your head and look again at your breasts (Diagram 2-3). Finally, press your hands against your hips and push inward, flexing your chest muscles as you inspect your breasts.

Look for any change in the skin, nipple, or areola since your last self-examination, including:
- changes in skin color
- skin swelling that stretches pores and makes them bigger, giving your skin the appearance of "orange peel"
- bumpiness that pushes the skin outward
- skin dimpling or indentation
- nipple crusting (dried nipple discharge) or actual discharge

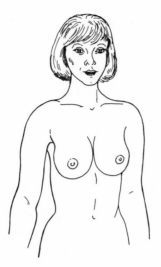

DIAGRAM 2-2   Inspection of the Breasts: With Arms Down

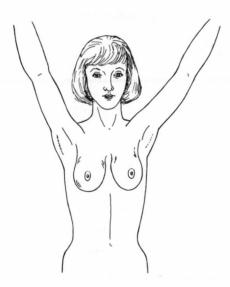

DIAGRAM 2-3   Inspection of the Breasts: With Arms Up

† PALPATION †

While palpating your breasts, look for any change since your last self-examination, including:

- a lump, soft or hard, that feels different from surrounding breast tissue
- a thickening of breast tissue which feels firmer than surrounding breast tissue
- thickening, puckering, or scaling of the skin or areola

What you might feel that *isn't* a problem:

- slight tenderness of part or all of a breast (many women have tender areas in their breasts); usually associated with fibrocystic changes (see Chapter 5)
- prominence of the ribs beneath the breast tissue
- a ridge of tissue (the "inframammary crease") on the underside of the breast where it attaches to the chest wall

STANDING OR SITTING

To palpate your right breast, position your right arm behind your head. Then, keeping the fingers of your left hand flat against the breast, press gently and systematically over its entire surface—either starting at the nipple and working outward in overlapping circles or starting at the top and working back and forth, then up and down, over the entire breast (Diagrams 2-4 and 2-5). Do the same thing again, using slightly stronger pressure. Now feel deep in the armpit for any lumps (Diagram 2-6). Reverse this procedure to palpate the left breast.

Many women feel their breasts in the shower, when their

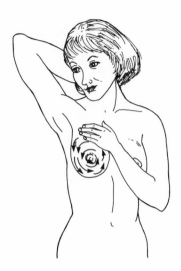

DIAGRAM 2-4   Palpation of the Breasts: Circular Method

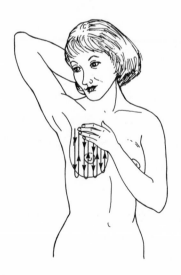

DIAGRAM 2-5   Palpation of the Breasts: Up-and-Down Method

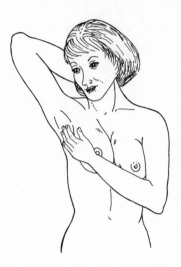

DIAGRAM 2-6   Palpation of the Armpit (Axilla):
Standing or Sitting

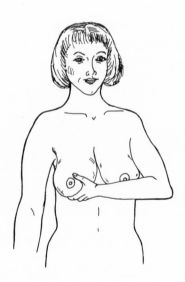

DIAGRAM 2-7   Palpation of Droopy Breasts: Standing or Sitting

breasts are wet and soapy and their fingers glide over them more easily.

If your breasts are somewhat droopy, you should also palpate them by placing your thumb in front and your fingers in back, then moving them around the entire breast (Diagram 2-7).

A word of caution: Use one technique or the other. Don't alternate. Remember, the point is to use an unvarying method for examining your breasts so that any changes from the previous examination will stand out clearly.

LYING DOWN

Lie down with a pillow or folded towel under your shoulder on the same side as the breast you'll be examining first. Then examine your breasts exactly as before. When you're lying down, with the breast tissue spread out and flattened over the chest wall, you can more easily detect any changes since your last self-examination. (Diagram 2-8.)

Finally, squeeze each nipple very gently. Does any liquid (discharge) seep out? If so, is it clear, greenish, or bloody? I recommend reporting *any* discharge to your doctor.

† WHICH DOCTOR SHOULD YOU CALL? †

These days, a woman can expect to have ongoing connections with several doctors—an internist or family physician, a gynecologist, a surgeon if you've had surgery or a surgical consultation in the recent past, and one or more other spe-

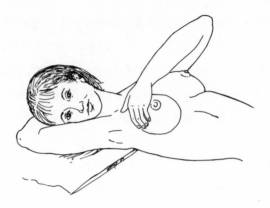

DIAGRAM 2-8   Palpation of the Breasts: Lying Down

cialists if you have any chronic health problems. Which one should you call? Here are a few guidelines:

- Whichever doctor you call, expect to receive an appointment to see him or her within a week. *Don't accept delays.*
- If you've never seen a surgeon for breast problems, call your internist, family physician, or gynecologist. (If you don't have a regular doctor, call your city or county medical society or your local hospital for a referral.)
- If you have previously seen a surgeon for breast problems, call that surgeon. After examining you, he or she will send a report to your internist or family physician.

† A FINAL WORD: OVERCOMING DENIAL †

If you do find a lump in your breast one day, how do you think you'll feel? If you're like most women, the discovery will momentarily stun you with the fear of breast cancer.

That's a perfectly understandable reaction. But sometimes that fear is so overwhelming a woman can't face the idea of making an appointment with her doctor until the lump has grown too large to ignore. By that time, if it's cancer, treatment is less likely to be completely successful.

Don't let denial paralyze your usual common sense. Instead, start coping by reminding yourself that *four out of five women with breast abnormalities do not have cancer.* They may have benign (fibrocystic) changes or they may have nothing at all. Those are pretty good odds. And for the one woman in five whose breast lump is cancerous, early detection through breast self-examination can be lifesaving.

Denial only adds to the emotional burden of a woman concerned about a change in her breast. Be good to yourself. If you find a lump, see your doctor right away for diagnosis and treatment, as you would for any condition that threatened your health. That way, you control your fear; it doesn't control you.

3

The Miracle of Mammography

It's a paradox: Although mammography saves many women's lives each year by finding their breast cancer at early and highly treatable stages, *only about 15 percent of women who should have regular mammograms actually do.* So although doctors now consider mammography indispensable in their fight against breast cancer, clearly most women are not yet convinced. Doctors initially were skeptical of the value of mammography, but huge studies such as the Breast Cancer Detection Demonstration Project, involving over 280,000 women, have proven its effectiveness beyond any doubt. Of 4,240 breast cancers detected in that study, 1,375 were found by mammography alone. That group of patients had the most successful treatment results. Had their cancers not been found by mammography, they would have continued to grow until they were large enough to be felt.[1]

A study from the Kaiser Permanente Medical Center has shown that cancers found by mammography alone had lymph node involvement only about half as often as those found by palpation. Treatment is much more successful if no lymph nodes contain cancer.[2]

Why is there such an enormous gap between doctors' and women's acceptance of mammography? In the course of examining many women and recommending that they have regular mammograms, I've heard a variety of responses:

- "I'm afraid mammography isn't safe—because it uses X-rays."
- "Mammography's too expensive!"
- "I'm not convinced mammography works all that well."
- "I've heard that finding a breast cancer early doesn't make any difference in whether treatment is successful or not."
- "It's too painful."
- "There has never been any breast cancer in my family."

Except for the fact that mammography is still fairly expensive (but increasingly covered by health insurance), *all these beliefs are either just plain wrong or dangerously outmoded.* Mammography *is* safe. It *is* worth the expense and effort involved. *Every* woman over 35 should follow a lifelong schedule for mammographic screening, and younger women at high risk for breast cancer should start even sooner (see Table 3-1).

Mrs. Beatrice LaRue, age 63, came to me after her first-ever screening mammogram. It showed a dominant one-centimeter (about one-half-inch) lump that the radiologist considered highly suspicious for cancer. The lump was not yet large enough to feel under the skin surface.

A biopsy confirmed the radiologist's suspicion, and Mrs. LaRue opted for treatment by lumpectomy with lymph node removal, followed by irradiation therapy. That was five years ago and she's had no recurrence of the cancer. If we hadn't found the lump at such an early stage, it would have continued to grow and might have involved the lymph nodes by the time it grew large enough to feel beneath the skin. At 63, she was lucky indeed: I've seen a number of women her age with advanced cancer that could not be completely eradicated—who also had not had regular screening mammograms.

Use the following recommendations from the American College of Radiology and the American Cancer Society to discuss and set up your personal mammography schedule with your doctor.

TABLE 3-1

Mammography Screening Schedule

Age Range	Mammography Recommendations
Up to 35	Not routinely recommended (incidence of breast cancer is low, women's breasts are more glandular and mammograms are more difficult to interpret) but the doctor may advise a mammogram based on evaluation of risk factors
35 to 39	Initial mammogram for comparison with future ones and detection of any current abnormalities
40 to 49	Mammogram every one or two years, depending on the doctor's evaluation of risk factors
50 and over	Screening mammogram yearly

† What Mammography Is †

Mammography is the process of taking an X-ray of the breast to detect any abnormalities. Whether taken in the doctor's office or a hospital, or in a mobile mammography van, all mammograms are reviewed by a radiologist (a specialist in evaluating X-ray examinations). She reports her findings to your doctor, or to you if the mammogram was taken without a doctor's referral.

Two types of mammography are used today: *film screen mammography*, which produces an image on X-ray film, and *xeromammography*, which produces a blue image against a white background on a piece of paper or cardboard. Radiologists say that both X-ray films and xeromammograms are equally "readable" and I agree; my patients may have either, depending on where the mammogram is done. (Most hospitals and clinics use one type or the other, not both.) (See Table 3-2.)

In 1989 the Xerox Corporation announced that it will no longer be producing xeromammographic equipment but will service existing equipment for at least five years. However, it is still being used in many places today.

† What Is It Like to Have † a Mammogram?

For convenience, the word *mammogram* is usually used to mean four to six X-ray views of your breasts, taken in quick succession.

TABLE 3-2

Types of Mammograms

Xeromammogram	X-Ray (Film) Mammogram
Uses slightly higher dose of irradiation	Uses smallest dose of irradiation
Requires less breast compression	Requires more breast compression
Produces a blue image on a white background on cardboard	Produces an X-ray film image
Uses specialized xerographic equipment for use only to image the breasts	Uses specialized X-ray equipment for use only to image the breasts
Images are easy to "read"	Images are slightly more difficult to "read"
"Reading" does not require an X-ray view box	"Reading" requires an X-ray view box

On the day of your mammogram, don't use any deodorant or powder in or near your underarms or breasts. For comfort and convenience, wear a blouse or sweater that will permit you to undress just from the waist up.

In the radiology department, your breasts may be examined before your mammogram is taken or you may be sent directly to the mammography area. You may be asked to sit, stand, or lie down for the procedure, depending on the type of equipment used. Each breast is rested on a firm surface and imaged separately while being compressed and held in position with a plastic shield, a balloon, or a sponge. Many women complain of some discomfort when their breasts are being compressed. But the benefits are well worth that discomfort and the compression is not harmful.

Usually a radiologist checks the X-rays immediately to see if any "retakes" are needed. If they are, the procedure will be repeated.

Your doctor will have the results of your mammogram within a day or two. Someone from her office should call you or the doctor may ask you to call her office. Either way, *be sure you find out the results*. Never assume that everything is all right if you don't hear from the doctor. If necessary call her office and keep calling until you have the results.

If your mammogram is normal, you may get the results from the doctor's receptionist. If you have questions, your doctor should be willing to discuss them with you. If an abnormality appears on your mammogram, your doctor will ask you to come to the office to discuss it or will refer you to another physician.

When you arrive at the hospital or clinic for a mammogram, take a moment to ask about the equipment and procedures the staff will use. If necessary, take a copy of Table 3-3 with you.

† WHAT MAMMOGRAPHY MAY FIND †

Mammography is the *best* way we have to find a breast cancer early. About half of the breast cancers I see are now

TABLE 3-3

Getting the Most Mammogram for Your Money

What's Needed	*Why It's Needed*
New equipment, used only for mammography	New equipment uses least amount of radiation and gives the best images
Low-dose irradiation (less than 1 rad)	Low dose minimizes risk of X-ray exposure
Explanation of what patient should do to cooperate with mammography staff	Maximum cooperation ensures efficient, accurate test
Imaging of the entire breast (on the mammogram, an edge of muscle should be visible around the breast)	Complete imaging ensures that no abnormality will be missed
At least two (sometimes three) views of each breast	Multiple views also ensure that no abnormality will be missed and will "see" any suspicious finding from two or more directions
"Reading" of the mammogram by a trained and experienced radiologist	Radiologist's training and experience contribute to accurate result of "reading"

first discovered by mammography. Most of these women and their physicians did not feel any abnormality in their breasts. Several findings are considered suspicious when detected by

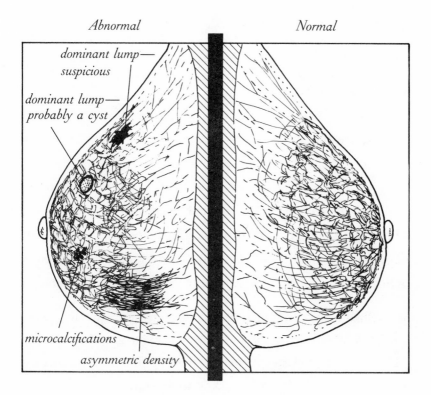

Abnormal   *Normal*

dominant lump—
suspicious

dominant lump—
probably a cyst

microcalcifications

asymmetric density

DIAGRAM 3-1   Mammogram

mammography: a dominant lump, a group of microcalcifications, and breast tissue asymmetry (Diagram 3-1).

DOMINANT LUMPS

A dominant lump appears different from the other tissue in
the breast. The most common abnormality detected by mammography, it can be any shape or size and may or may not
be cancerous. Fibrocystic changes that take the form of dominant lumps (such as cysts or fibroadenomas) usually appear
more rounded than cancers, which are typically more irregular.

Only an aspiration or biopsy can tell for sure if a dominant lump is a cyst, some other benign condition, or cancer.

MICROCALCIFICATIONS

These tiny flecks of calcium, seen in the soft tissues of the breasts, are the second most common abnormality noted on mammograms. Some types are associated with fibrocystic changes, others with cancer. The most suspicious microcalcifications are clustered together in one small area in the breast. These must always be biopsied. Much less worrisome are larger microcalcifications scattered throughout one or both breasts; most often, these represent only fibrocystic changes.

Mrs. Roberta Anthony, age 38, came to see me after her latest screening mammogram showed a tiny five-millimeter (one-quarter inch in diameter) clustered area of microcalcifications located very close to the nipple. It was too small to feel through the skin, so I had to perform a needle localization and biopsy, which indicated that she had an intraductal cancer. She decided to have a lumpectomy, followed by breast irradiation. Cancer had not spread beyond the duct, so lymph node involvement would not be expected. Because mammography found her cancer early, I consider her chances of recurrence to be almost nil—less than 2 percent.

BREAST TISSUE ASYMMETRY

As imaged on a mammogram, "asymmetrical" breast tissue appears denser or distorted compared with the surrounding tissues or with the same location in the other breast. This is one of the most variable and difficult changes to "read" in a mammogram, since every woman has some differences in the appearance of the X-rays of each breast. Mammography may also reveal such suspicious findings as skin thickening, prominence of one or more ducts, or nipple retraction.

† How Safe Is Mammography? †

Today's state-of-the-art mammography equipment uses less than 1 rad (unit of irradiation)—often less than ½ rad—to image the breast. Even repeated for thirty to forty years, at this low dosage mammography carries no risk. The dosage is lower than was possible just a few years ago and the images are even better. Some older units are still in operation, however, so when you have a mammogram, ask if the equipment meets the latest standards for low-dosage irradiation.

The safety of mammography is based on more than just conjecture. There simply has never been a proven case of mammography-induced breast cancer. That explains why mammography has the full and enthusiastic endorsement of the American Cancer Society, the American College of Radiology, the American College of Surgeons, and the Food and Drug Administration.

† Comparing New and Old Mammograms †

Whenever possible, each mammogram you have should be compared with the previous one(s). Sometimes with the help of such a comparison it is possible to prove that a somewhat suspicious area on a woman's most recent mammogram was actually present one or two years earlier. With newer equipment, it just shows up more clearly. If it was present then and if it hasn't changed size or shape, we know it needs no further investigation. Cancers do not stay the same for a year; only benign changes remain static.

Of course, if a woman hasn't had a mammogram before, or if she's had some but can't obtain them for review, then any suspicious finding must be investigated thoroughly.

Ms. Claudia Emile, age 36, came to see me recently for a second surgeon's opinion of a benign-appearing asymmetrical area of thickened breast tissue in the upper and outer portion of her right breast seen only on mammography. I reviewed the mammogram taken just a few days before. I then discovered that she had had mammography performed at another hospital three years earlier. We had a messenger service pick up those films. I showed those to the radiologist in our hospital, who agreed that the area appeared identical in both mammograms except that the three-year-old mammogram was not of the same quality. These findings proved that the asymmetry was normal and she would need no treatment, only routine screening.

† OTHER USES OF MAMMOGRAPHY †
MAMMOGRAPHY BEFORE BIOPSY

Even when a lump is big enough for your doctor to feel, she should recommend that you have a mammogram before a biopsy. The mammogram may reveal additional suspicious areas, in either breast, that can be biopsied at the same time as the original lump.

After Mrs. Adriana Angelina, age 45, found a lump in her left breast, a pre-biopsy mammogram showed another, much smaller lump in her right breast. I biopsied both lumps at the same time and found ductal hyperplasia, a benign fibrocystic change, on the left—but cancer on the right. Without that mammogram, the cancerous lump in the right breast would have continued to grow and might possibly have invaded lymph node tissue by the time it was discovered. Three years after her treatment, Mrs. Angelina has no evidence of any cancer. And because it was discovered early, I expect her to continue to do well.

IS A LUMP SUSPICIOUS?

Mammography is also used to help confirm the presence of a questionable lump found during the doctor's examination.

Ms. Connie Jackson, age 39, noted a "lump" in her right breast. When I examined her, the area of concern was thickened and different from the other side, but I couldn't feel a definite lump. I was not very concerned and considered it quite safe to watch this and see her in a month. But to provide an added measure of support for my decision, I ordered a mammogram. It showed no abnormality. The following month the "lump" was no longer evident; it had only been a fibrocystic change.

NEEDLE LOCALIZATION

Mammography is frequently used to locate a suspicious area (previously detected on a screening mammogram) so that the surgeon can find the correct tissue to biopsy. Known as "needle localization and biopsy," the use of this technique has increased more than tenfold in the past four years. (Diagrams 3-2 and 3-3.)

To undergo needle localization you are seated in front of

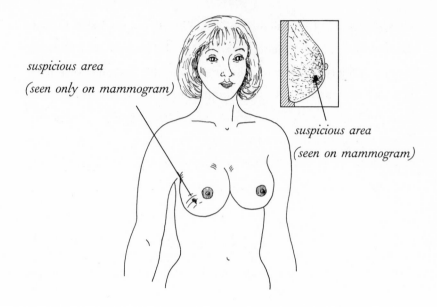

suspicious area
(seen only on mammogram)

suspicious area
(seen on mammogram)

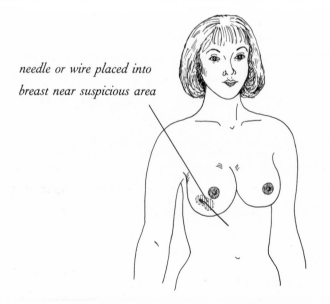

needle or wire placed into
breast near suspicious area

DIAGRAMS 3-2 and 3-3   Needle Localization

the mammography unit and a small amount of local anesthesia is injected into the skin of the breast. Then a needle or wire is inserted into the breast near the suspicious area and gently moved very close to it while one or more mammograms are taken. With the needle still in place, you are taken to the operating room, where the surgeon uses the location of the needle on the mammograms to plan the biopsy incision.

Following the needle down to the suspicious area, the surgeon removes that tissue. To verify that he has removed the targeted area, he frequently sends the specimen to be X-rayed. If it is the tissue he intended to remove, it will look the same on this X-ray as it did on the mammogram. If it doesn't, the surgeon will have to remove more tissue and repeat the X-ray verification until he is sure the entire suspicious area is removed.

When Ms. Sara Thomas, age 45, had her first screening mammogram, it showed a dominant lump in her left breast. A centimeter in diameter, with clustered microcalcifications, it was very suspicious for cancer. I couldn't feel it, because her breasts were large and it was deep. So I recommended a needle localization and biopsy, which took place the next day. Fortunately, like so many suspicious mammograhic findings, it proved to be a fibrocystic change—sclerosing adenosis.

DUCTOGRAM

Used to examine abnormal nipple discharge, a ductogram requires the radiologist and surgeon to work closely together. The surgeon determines the exact location of the draining

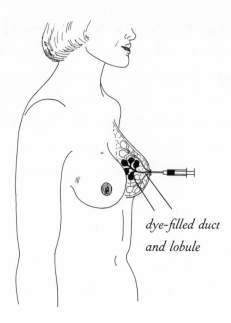

*dye-filled duct
and lobule*

DIAGRAM 3-4   Ductogram

duct. The radiologist inserts a tiny, blunt needle into that duct
and injects a small amount of dye that can be seen on a
mammogram. A mammogram is then taken for two purposes:
first, to outline the entire suspicious lobule, and second, to
determine if a small polyp or other abnormality is seen in any
of the ducts visualized. Then a colored dye is injected so the
surgeon can more easily find the suspicious area. This test is
best performed just prior to the biopsy. (Diagram 3-4.)

† WHAT MAMMOGRAPHY CAN'T DO—YET †

Mammography is our most valuable tool for pinpointing
suspicious areas in the breast; it is hoped that in the future it

will be able to indicate whether a lump is cancerous or not as well.

At present we must biopsy any suspicious mass found by mammography, even though about 80 percent of breast lumps turn out to be benign. When and if mammography becomes capable of differentiating cancerous areas from normal ones, fewer women will undergo biopsy of benign breast tissue.

† When Mammography May † Not Be Needed

Twenty-one-year-old Ms. JoAnne Eller came to see me because of a one-centimeter (half-inch) lump she'd found in the lower portion of her right breast. I suspected it was a benign lump, probably a fibroadenoma, and I recommended that she have a biopsy *without* having a mammogram first. In a woman so young, breast tissue is very dense (a hindrance to mammography) and breast cancer is extremely rare. The biopsy confirmed my original impression; the lump was a fibroadenoma.

† Knowledge Is Power †

"Health and fitness" is a way of life for many women today. They watch their weight, they know their cholesterol count, maybe even their pulse rates at rest and during exercise. And thanks to mammography, increasing numbers of them know for sure how healthy their breasts are.

That kind of knowledge gives you power, the power to plan your life instead of waiting for what may or may not happen and then reacting to it. If you're over 35, plan to have regular mammograms. They're available and affordable, and they're saving more women's lives than ever before.

WILL NEW BREAST-IMAGING TECHNIQUES REPLACE MAMMOGRAPHY?

Techniques besides mammography have been proposed for detecting tissue changes in the breasts, including thermography, computer tomography (CT) imaging, transillumination, ultrasound, and magnetic resonance imaging (MRI). So far, *none of them can do what mammography does*; its image quality remains unsurpassed.

Thermography, which evaluates changes in the breasts' skin temperature, is not recommended by the American College of Radiology. After studying thermography for years with little or no positive results, most researchers have concluded that cancers "found" by thermography were in fact found by chance—usually when a lump was already big enough to feel. Because thermography has none of the capabilities of mammography and offers no unique advantage, I don't use it or recommend it for my patients. It's a waste of time and money.

CT imaging, a recently developed form of X-ray, is still under investigation for breast screening. So far, it stacks up poorly against mammography. It may require injection of intravenous contrast material, and it offers few or no clues to differentiating between fibrocystic and cancerous breast changes. It is also very expensive; an examination costs hundreds of dollars.

Transillumination, shining strong light through the breast to highlight internal structures, is also experimental at this time. It typically misses four out of five breast lumps less than one centimeter (one-half inch) in diameter and even one of every four lumps larger than two centimeters (one inch) in diameter.

Ultrasound (sonography), a technique that produces an X-ray-like image by sending sound waves into the body and "reading" them as they bounce back off body structures, is frequently used to supplement mammography—but never to replace it. Ultrasound can differentiate solid from liquid areas in the breast, so it's very helpful in detecting cysts and localizing them for aspiration. But because it has little capacity to detect small breast lumps or to suggest that a lump may or may not be cancerous, ultrasound is not a substitute for mammography.

Her first screening mammogram revealed that Mrs. Jackie Flora, age 40, had a smooth, round dominant mass in the center of her breast. I could not feel it. The radiologist and I, working closely together, performed an ultrasound examination and determined that the lump was a fluid-filled cyst. Using the ultrasound screen, a small hypodermic needle was guided into the cyst, the fluid was removed, and the cyst disappeared. Without the guidance of ultrasound, Mrs. Flora would have needed a biopsy.

Magnetic resonance imaging, a new procedure that uses no irradiation and can find lumps in even very dense breast tissue, may have a future role in screening for breast changes. So far, it's also experimental—and it remains extremely expensive.

4

Diagnosing the Problem:
Breast Biopsy

Mammography and physical examination screen for evidence of possible breast problems; breast biopsy provides the diagnosis. In this minor surgical procedure, the surgeon removes either all of the abnormal breast tissue or, in some cases, a small piece of it. Then a pathologist examines its cells under the microscope.

† WHAT ARE THE SUSPICIOUS FINDINGS †
THAT WILL LEAD TO BIOPSY?

Dominant mass or asymmetric density. A biopsy is most commonly prompted by a lump or thickening in the breast. The woman may have found it herself, by accident or during self-examination, or her doctor may find it while examining her breasts by palpation or by mammography.

Microcalcifications. These dots of calcium in the breast tissue (as small as 1/32nd of an inch in diameter but sometimes slightly larger), clustered together in a small area, can be seen only on a mammogram. They may or may not be surrounded by a dominant mass.

Nipple discharge. Many women on occasion have a clear discharge from both nipples; this is rarely a problem. What does raise a doctor's suspicions is any bloody drainage or a nonbloody one if it is coming from only one nipple.

If a woman has any type of suspicious finding in her breast, she will want to know her diagnosis as quickly as possible, and she should have a biopsy sometime in the next few days.

† Is It Cancer? †

During our preliminary discussion, my patients almost always ask me, "Do you think it's cancer?" In this situation, I don't make the diagnosis—the biopsy will do that. So I'm not going to make a possibly upsetting (or wrong) guess either. What I can usually say with confidence is that statistics are generally on my patient's side. Although the risk of breast cancer depends on a woman's age (see Table 4-1), approximately four out of five biopsies identify *noncancerous* conditions.

TABLE 4-1

Incidence of Breast Cancer in Women of
Varying Ages, as Revealed by Biopsy

Age	Percent of Biopsies That Find Cancer
Under 40	10 to 15%
40 to 49	20 to 25%
50 to 59	30 to 35%
60 and over	40 to 50%

† The Next Step †

When a suspicious area is found in a woman's breast, she and her doctor should discuss the need for a biopsy. If she is over 30, a mammogram should be ordered. If the lump or thickening is found by physical examination and appears to be only a fibrocystic change, her doctor may elect to wait and watch the problem through one menstrual cycle. It is safe to wait this short period of time, but I never wait much longer before deciding whether or not to do a biopsy. Early treatment of breast cancer is critical.

In my experience, few patients have refused to have an outpatient biopsy once I've explained that we need to investigate a suspicious finding. No surgery should be taken lightly, but a biopsy is truly a limited procedure that carries almost no risk of adverse effects.

† Understanding the Types of Breast Biopsies †

Because breast biopsy is a type of surgery, I always explain to my patient in detail why it's necessary, what's involved in having it, and what we can expect to learn from it. Here's an overview of the types of biopsies most in use today.

MOST COMMON: Excisional Biopsy (Diagrams 4-1 and 4-1A)

Most breast biopsies are *excisional*—that is, the surgeon removes the entire area of abnormal breast tissue. That way, all the abnormal tissue is available for microscopic examination. Although this is the most extensive biopsy procedure, it can almost always be done on an outpatient basis using only local anesthesia.

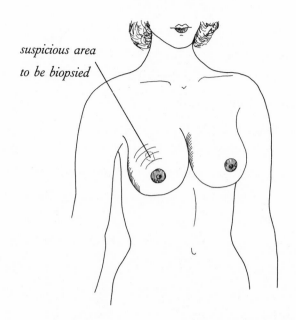

suspicious area to be biopsied

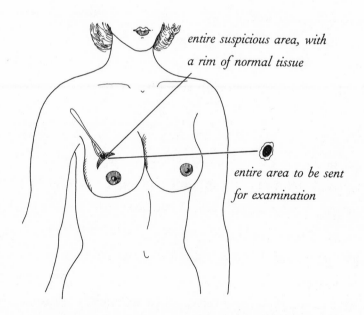

entire suspicious area, with a rim of normal tissue

entire area to be sent for examination

DIAGRAMS 4-1 and 4-1A   Excisional Biopsy

If a cancerous condition is diagnosed, this complete sample allows the pathologist to identify all the cancer's characteristics so the surgeon can plan comprehensive treatment. More commonly, a noncancerous condition is diagnosed, for which no further treatment is necessary.

There is now another advantage to excisional biopsy. If cancer is found and if the surgeon was able during the biopsy to remove a rim of normal tissue with the cancer, the patient would have completed the lumpectomy part of a breast-conservation procedure. (See Chapter 9.) A lumpectomy is essentially a large biopsy.

LESS COMMON: NEEDLE-CORE BIOPSY (DIAGRAM 4-2)

The doctor uses a special needle to remove a cylindrical core of the abnormal breast tissue, about the thickness of the lead of a wood pencil. Although this type of biopsy is simpler than the others (it requires no incision), it removes only a small amount of tissue and may give an incomplete picture of the problem area. This office procedure requires no preparation by the patient or the surgeon. It can be decided upon and performed immediately, even during the first office visit. It's used mainly to confirm cancer in large or highly suspicious lumps. If needle-core biopsy does reveal cancer, no other biopsy is needed. The entire lump will be removed during the primary surgical procedure selected to treat the cancer. If cancer is not found in that sampling, the entire suspicious area should nonetheless be removed by excisional biopsy to make sure that cancer is present nowhere in the suspicious area.

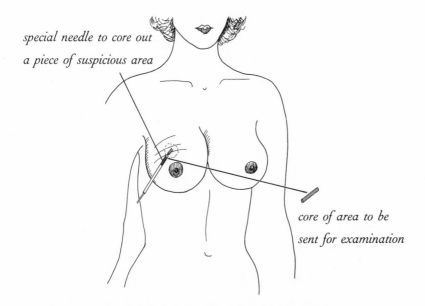

special needle to core out
a piece of suspicious area

core of area to be
sent for examination

DIAGRAM 4-2   Needle-Core Biopsy

LESS COMMON: INCISIONAL BIOPSY (DIAGRAM 4-3)

Like needle-core biopsy, which is gradually replacing it, incisional biopsy is used mainly to investigate large, highly suspicious breast lumps. The surgeon removes only a sliver or a small piece of the abnormal tissue through a small cut in the breast, and this piece is examined under the microscope. As with a needle-core biopsy, if cancer is not found, the patient will need an excisional biopsy to remove the entire suspicious area.

LEAST COMMON: MULTIPLE-NEEDLE ASPIRATION

In this procedure a needle and syringe are used to withdraw tissue cells from a lump for laboratory analysis. This method

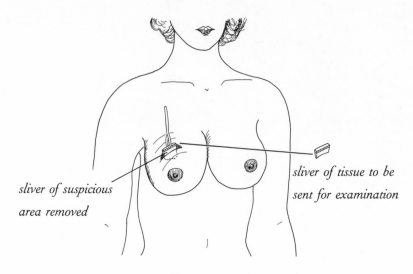

sliver of suspicious area removed

sliver of tissue to be sent for examination

DIAGRAM 4-3   Incisional Biopsy

removes only a small amount of tissue; usually an open biopsy is still needed if cancer is found, before treatment is begun. For this reason, multiple-needle aspiration is considered experimental at this time.

Extensive studies at the University of Wisconsin have shown that multiple-needle aspiration is helpful in confirming what are already considered to be nonsuspicious findings so biopsy can be avoided, or in proving that cancer is present.[1] Its final use is still unknown at this time.

† NEEDLE LOCALIZATION AND BIOPSY †
USING MAMMOGRAPHY

If a lump and/or microcalcifications are discovered by mammography, the doctor usually can't feel the suspicious area under the skin surface. In this situation, she'll probably do a needle localization before the biopsy, the only way to locate such an abnormality deep within the breast tissue. Using the needle or wire as a guide, the surgeon will plan the incision in such a way that the suspicious area within the breast can be readily found and removed by excisional biopsy. (See page 56.)

† Biopsy for Abnormal Nipple Discharge †

If the biopsy is being done to explore the cause of abnormal nipple discharge, the doctor usually can't feel a lump *or* see any abnormalities on a mammogram. The surest way to identify what is causing the discharge is to perform a special X-ray examination called a ductogram. (See page 49.) The surgeon can then find the abnormal duct and lobule and remove it by excisional biopsy.

Occasionally the involved duct can't be located. Then the doctor may remove a cylindrical core of tissue, about half an inch thick, from beneath the areola. Typically, this tissue contains the source of the discharge.

† Choosing a Biopsy Procedure †

Today, few women are hospitalized for breast biopsies. Biopsy is usually done in the hospital on an outpatient basis, following either the "one step" or the "two step" procedure.

The "One Step" Procedure

This procedure includes both the biopsy and the treatment for the cancer if it is found. Some women prefer to "get it over with" if the biopsy reveals cancer. The woman and her surgeon discuss her situation thoroughly to decide on her treatment. Then she has a biopsy under general rather than local anesthesia, so that, if cancer is found, the surgeon can proceed with whatever operation they had decided upon during their discussion(s). With this "one step" procedure, the woman doesn't know whether she has cancer or not until she wakes from anesthesia.

THE "TWO STEP" PROCEDURE

Today, most women elect to follow the "two step" procedure. The first step is the biopsy; only local anesthesia is needed, and the woman spends no more than a few hours in the hospital. Then, if the biopsy reveals breast cancer, the woman and her doctor take time to obtain additional tests (if needed to determine the extent of the cancer), to discuss treatment methods, and to get an oncologist's and/or a second surgeon's opinion.

PROS AND CONS

Four out of five women who have breast biopsies turn out *not* to have cancer. So four out of five women who elect the "one step" biopsy procedure unnecessarily experience the anguish of discussing treatment options for cancer they probably don't have. They also unnecessarily incur the cost of general anesthesia and the slight risk of adverse effects associated with it. Therefore the "one step" procedure is used less often now. (I have used it only rarely in the last 500 biopsies I've performed.)

Furthermore, although the preliminary (pre-biopsy) discussions allow the woman to express her treatment preferences generally, chances are the surgeon may have to make some crucial decisions during the surgery—decisions the woman can't participate in.

The "two step" procedure gives the woman a much greater role in planning her own treatment. It also allows time for her to prepare herself emotionally and to make arrangements for her care during recovery. Studies show that this brief delay in starting treatment does nothing to jeopardize the chance that it will be successful.

† What Happens During Breast Biopsy? †

Prior to the "one step" procedure, you will be required to sign an operative permit or consent form, not only for the biopsy but also for the operation you have previously agreed to should cancer be found. The surgeon performs the biopsy and gives the tissue he's removed to the pathologist for immediate analysis. Within twenty minutes, while the woman is still under anesthesia, the diagnosis is known. If the tissue isn't cancerous, the surgeon closes the biopsy and the woman can usually return home the same day. If cancer is present, the doctor performs the surgery in accordance with his previous discussions with his patient.

The "two step" procedure is scheduled on an outpatient basis. You can expect to spend up to three hours in the hospital on the appointed day, and you will be asked to sign an operative permit only for the biopsy. To biopsy a lump he can feel, the surgeon swabs the breast with an antiseptic solution, injects a local anesthetic (this is minimally painful), and waits briefly for it to take effect. Then he performs the biopsy.

This is *minor* surgery. You will feel some pulling and a sense of pressure, but no sharp pain. (If you do feel sharp pain, tell the doctor; he'll inject more of the local anesthetic.)

The doctor gives the tissue specimen to the waiting pathologist, who will prepare it for microscopic examination. And you're ready to leave the hospital. (Be sure to make a follow-up appointment with your doctor for one or two days hence.)

Depending on the type of material used to close the skin where the biopsy was done, you may also be asked to make an appointment for suture removal about a week after the procedure.

† Your Follow-up Visit to the Doctor †

When you see your doctor to discuss the biopsy results, chances are you'll learn that the biopsy has removed the cause of your breast problem. If you do have cancer, your doctor should spend up to an hour with you, giving you time to absorb the diagnosis and then discussing your treatment options with you in detail.

† To Biopsy or Not: The Need † for a Second Opinion

Mrs. Jane Myrick, age 53, came to see me for my opinion on whether she should have a breast biopsy. She'd never had any problem with her breasts, and three years earlier a screening mammogram had shown no abnormalities. But her latest mammogram did show a change: a dominant mass, deep in her left breast, that could not yet be felt.

Her own doctor sent her to a surgeon for his opinion; he recommended needle localization and excisional biopsy. Then she consulted another surgeon, who did *not* think the lump was suspicious. He recommended that she wait six months and then have another mammogram to see if the lump had changed. Which recommendation should she follow? She opted for one more surgical opinion: mine.

Certainly Mrs. Myrick didn't want to have unnecessary surgery— a topic much in the news these days. But she knew the importance of finding out what the lump in her breast meant. After reviewing all her mammograms with our radiologist, I agreed with the first surgeon that her lump should be biopsied without delay. The first surgeon performed the needle localization and excisional biopsy— which revealed an early intraductal cancer.

What would have happened if she'd taken the second surgeon's advice and waited six months before having another mammogram? The cancer might still have been located entirely within the duct, but it might also have begun to spread into the breast and beyond. Happily, with treatment at this early stage, her prognosis was excellent.

5

Most Lumps Aren't Cancer: Understanding Fibrocystic Changes

Lumpy breasts, cystic disease, and *mastitis* are terms popularly used to describe the many noncancerous breast conditions that affect half of all women in North America. Unfortunately, they are more confusing and frightening than informative.

Doctors use the term *fibrocystic changes* or, erroneously, *fibrocystic disease.* Most of these changes are variations of normal tissues, so they aren't really diseases. Lumpy fibrocystic changes can arise anywhere in breast tissue—glands, ducts, or fibrous tissue.

Almost every woman I see in my office either has some type of fibrocystic change in her breasts (usually a mix of types) or has been told she has. Like most people, you've probably heard rumors about fibrocystic changes—that they lead to cancer, for example. This misinformation creates needless anxiety. The vast majority of fibrocystic changes *aren't* cancer. They rarely increase a woman's risk of breast cancer, and they usually require *little or no treatment.*

Unfortunately, finding a lump or other breast change almost always raises the specter of cancer in a woman's mind, overshadowing the much greater likelihood that if she has a problem at all, it's a fibrocystic change. Over and over again, I've examined women who waited weeks or months before coming in and suffered painful anxiety in the interim, only to learn that their fears of cancer were groundless.

† CONTROLLING CANCER FEARS †

When you discover a change in your breasts' feel or contour, remember three things:

1. A doctor's examination and a mammogram provide the best and quickest way to get control of your fear.

2. Fibrocystic changes are *not* breast cancer and your risk of developing breast cancer after having most types of fibrocystic changes is no greater than that in women without fibrocystic changes.

3. Of the multitude of fibrocystic changes that can occur, only two less common ones—atypical ductal hyperplasia and ductal papillomatosis—have *any* association with the development of breast cancer. And even then, the increased risk is small. Only a minor percentage of women with these changes will actually develop cancer.

If fibrocystic changes don't usually cause breast cancer, why are women afraid of them? Not so long ago, doctors thought that all women with fibrocystic "disease" had an increased risk of breast cancer. This naturally heightened cancer fears in the large population of women who developed fibrocystic changes in their breasts.

Now doctors have identified the various fibrocystic changes

and studied them individually, so we can reassure concerned women that the overwhelming majority of these changes are completely noncancerous. Because so many women have fibrocystic changes, one out of ten will eventually develop breast cancer—the same percentage as in the general population; but the two events are almost never related.

† Who Gets Fibrocystic Changes? †

Certain personal characteristics (risk factors) may boost a woman's likelihood of developing fibrocystic changes, but not by much. The general risk (30 to 50 percent) is already quite high. Surveys show that women who are small-breasted and thin are somewhat more likely to develop fibrocystic changes, but it may simply be that because their breasts have less fatty tissue, the diagnosis is easier to make than in heavier women.

Mrs. Alice Howard, age 30, had never had any complaints characteristic of fibrocystic changes but now felt numerous lumpy areas in her breasts. My examination was puzzlingly inconclusive until I asked her if she'd recently lost weight. "Why, yes, forty pounds!" she exclaimed, and the mystery was solved. The extra fatty tissue in her breasts had previously masked the normal glandular structure, which she could now feel because of her weight loss.

Most fibrocystic breast changes develop during women's reproductive years, the decades between puberty and menopause. (After menopause, they occur much less often.) Certain fibrocystic changes are age-related. For example, young women have the highest incidence of fibroadenomas.

Fibrocystic changes are also slightly more common if the woman:

* never took oral contraceptives
* had an abortion
* takes estrogen for menopause symptoms
* has irregular menstrual cycles
* has a mother or sister with fibrocystic breast changes

† Is Caffeine a Risk Factor? †

In 1979, a group of doctors conducting studies of breast changes in women began to link caffeine with development of fibrocystic change.[1] When they asked women with fibrocystic changes to discontinue the use of coffee, cola drinks, and chocolate, the women reported the resolution of breast lumps and pain. When they resumed ingestion of those items, the problems recurred.

Foods and beverages that contain large amounts of caffeine are staples in the American diet, so this indictment of caffeine was news. Soon women (and doctors) everywhere believed that avoiding caffeine would help prevent fibrocystic changes or lessen the discomfort they cause.

More recently other studies have contradicted those findings by discovering no association between fibrocystic change and the use of caffeine.[2]

Today, doctors generally agree that no definite proof exists to support a connection. If you have fibrocystic changes and feel some concern about drinking coffee or eating chocolate, check with your doctor. He'll probably tell you what I tell my patients: Consuming less caffeine can't do you any harm and may even benefit your general health, but it isn't likely to relieve your breast discomfort.

† Symptoms of Fibrocystic Changes †

PAIN

Evaluating a woman's breast pain is never easy, because everyone experiences pain differently. However, pain in the breast usually points to fibrocystic changes. This appears to be caused by hormonal changes during the woman's menstrual cycle, worsening just before her period begins.

If the pain is so severe that it interferes with the woman's daily activities, I usually recommend nonprescription pain relievers (aspirin and the multitude of nonaspirin competitors). Among my patients I've also noticed that oral contraceptives have reduced breast pains, so they can occasionally be prescribed for that purpose. I *never* give a woman a prescription for a narcotic pain reliever, such as codeine, to treat ongoing breast pain. The danger of addiction is just too great.

In extremely rare cases of disabling breast pain (about five women so far in my entire practice), I've prescribed a medication called danazol, which reduces the body's production of estrogen and progesterone. Studies have shown that over 60 percent of women receiving danazol have diminished symptoms of fibrocystic change.[3] It can, however, have potentially severe side effects, including hormonal imbalance, acne, fluid retention, weight gain, and menstrual irregularities, so it must be used sparingly and carefully.

Diuretics ("water pills"), vitamin E, and special diets have been shown to have no effect on breast pain. Surgically removing a portion of the breast for pain is never done. It doesn't work. The painful fibrocystic changes simply recur elsewhere in the breast.

LUMPINESS

When I examine a woman's breasts and find a lump or lumpy area, I always explain what I've found and describe it using specific terms, such as *diffuse* or *dominant*. I don't use general terms, such as *mastitis* or *cystitis*. They may be misleading and they don't describe the lumpiness itself.

In many women I examine who turn out to have fibrocystic changes, I find a general (diffuse) feeling of lumpiness in one or both breasts. When this happens, I'm frequently able to tell my patient she needs no treatment at all. A dominant lump, however—one that feels separate from the surrounding tissue—needs further investigation. (Diagrams 5-1 and 5-2.)

If your doctor finds an area of lumpiness when he examines your breasts, ask whether it's diffuse or dominant. If it's dominant and he doesn't recommend further treatment or testing, consider getting a second opinion.

NIPPLE DISCHARGE

Secretion of fluid from the breast through the nipple can be annoying. A woman may notice it as a drop of fluid or

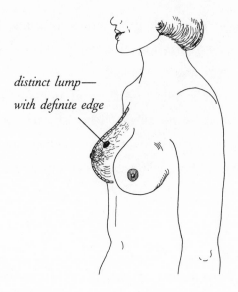

distinct lump—
with definite edge

DIAGRAM 5-1   Discrete Dominant Lump

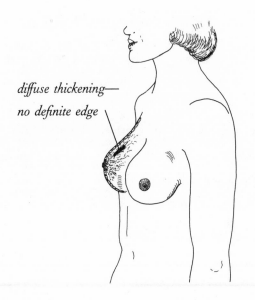

diffuse thickening—
no definite edge

DIAGRAM 5-2   Nondiscrete, Diffuse Lumpiness

crust of dried fluid on her nipple—or as a stain on her clothing directly over the nipple.

If the discharge is clear and occurs in both breasts, it's not usually a cause for concern. Most often it comes from ducts stretched by fibrocystic changes. However, clear or milky discharge from one breast, or any bloody discharge or discharge that occurs along with a breast lump, calls for a doctor's examination and, frequently, a biopsy. It often, but not always, indicates only fibrocystic changes.

† UNDERSTANDING FIBROCYSTIC CHANGES †

CYSTS

Cysts are breast glands and ducts that have filled with fluid in response to hormonal stimulation, stretched, and then ruptured together, forming a fluid-filled dominant lump that may be painful. They can feel smooth or rough, hard as a marble or softer. Sometimes they can't be felt but are visible on a mammogram. They may grow to a very large size and contain up to an ounce of fluid, but usually they're discovered and aspirated before this happens. Once aspirated, many cysts don't refill with fluid, but a significant number do. New cysts may later form in the same area of the breast or in different areas.

To reassure a woman that a dominant lump is a cyst, I aspirate it using local anesthesia when it is first noted. If it's filled with fluid, it disappears. As a final test, I will examine her again in about a month to make sure the lump hasn't reappeared. (Diagram 5-3.)

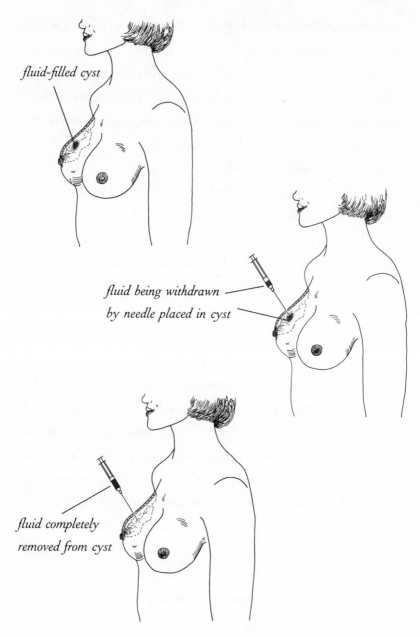

fluid-filled cyst

fluid being withdrawn
by needle placed in cyst

fluid completely
removed from cyst

DIAGRAM 5-3   Aspiration of a Cyst

What if the fluid withdrawn from a cyst is bloody, or if it does reappear within a few weeks? Popular belief has it that this may mean a cancer is growing in or near the cyst. *I have never had a single case like this*, although colleagues have reported a few. But to be on the safe side, I do a biopsy if the aspiration is bloody or if the cyst recurs after a few aspirations.

When Mrs. Joan Korwin, age 42, found three lumps in her right breast, she was understandably concerned. My examination indicated that the lumps were almost certainly cysts, but because she'd never had a mammogram, I asked her to have one before I aspirated them. Aspiration can sometimes cause very mild bleeding in the breast that creates false readings on mammograms for a number of days.

The mammogram showed the three large cysts plus some generalized fibrocystic changes and several tiny cysts. Nothing needed to be done about the smaller cysts. The three large cysts disappeared after I aspirated them and were still absent at her checkup a month later and at six-month checkups over the course of the next two years. Then a cyst appeared in the same area of her breast, I aspirated it, and, again, it never recurred. This pattern will probably continue. Although annoying, it poses no risk to Mrs. Korwin's health.

Adenosis

Adenosis is a solid dominant lump or an area of lumpiness that forms when breast glands multiply and grow together. If these particular lumps contain small amounts of calcium— visible on a mammogram—the condition is called *sclerosing adenosis*. The lump, which may be very firm, may or may not be painful. Because these dominant lumps can feel like a cancer, and may even look like cancer on a mammogram, a biopsy is the only way to be certain they aren't.

When I examined Mrs. Barbara George, age 50, I'd already seen her latest mammogram, which showed not only the lump in her breast but also several microcalcifications within it. These findings were rather suspicious, so I scheduled her for a biopsy—which indicated that the lump was a sclerosing adenosis. Once it was removed and we learned it wasn't cancerous, she needed no further treatment.

DUCTAL HYPERPLASIA

Like adenosis, *ductal hyperplasia* may take the form of a dominant lump, diffuse lumpiness, a cluster of microcalcifications visible on a mammogram, or a combination of these characteristics. It may or may not be painful. In *ductal ectasia*, a form of ductal hyperplasia, the ducts are filled with fluid and may cause pain and nipple discharge. If a dominant lump or any of certain types of nipple discharge is present, then a biopsy is required to be sure of the diagnosis. Although the duct tissue has formed a lump, when examined under a microscope the individual cells retain their normal appearance. (Diagram 5-4.)

If the cells develop an abnormal appearance, that's *atypical ductal hyperplasia*. Even though this abnormality is not breast cancer, studies show that women with this change develop

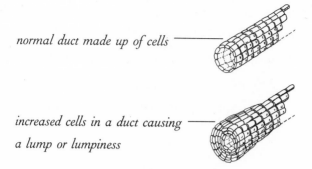

normal duct made up of cells

increased cells in a duct causing a lump or lumpiness

DIAGRAM 5-4   Ductal Hyperplasia

breast cancer more frequently. Apparently some connection does exist.

DUCTAL PAPILLOMATOSIS

Ductal papillomatosis occurs when the cells of one or more breast ducts grow into small painless polyps, called papillomas. These are attached to the duct walls (Diagram 5-5) and secrete blood or fluid that may be discharged from the nipple. Although one or many ducts may be affected, most—but not

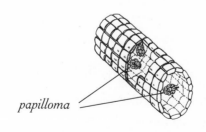

papilloma

DIAGRAM 5-5   Papillomas Inside a Duct

all—are too small to be felt or even seen on a mammogram. So a ductogram and a biopsy are needed to make the diagnosis.

Like atypical ductal hyperplasia, ductal papillomatosis is associated with a somewhat increased risk of breast cancer. A woman with this fibrocystic change should maintain constant vigilance.

When Ms. Jeanette Roland, age 40, discovered a small amount of blood on the bodice of her nightgown, she gave it little thought, assuming she must have scratched herself. She noticed it again a week or so later, and this time the spot was directly over her right breast. More blood came out when she squeezed the nipple. Alarmed, she made an immediate appointment with her gynecologist, who ordered a mammogram and then referred her to me.

The mammogram was normal. But I noticed that when I pressed one particular area on her right breast, the nipple discharged blood. Probably one duct of a single lobule was bleeding. Ductograms were not routinely used at that time, so I biopsied the area, making an incision around the areola to ensure miminal scarring. I found the blood-filled duct and removed the entire lobule for microscopic examination in the laboratory. Several papillomas were discovered, all noncancerous.

FIBROSIS

Fibrosis is simply an overgrowth of the fibrous (connective) tissue surrounding the breast glands. It can occur anytime but is most common following the onset of menopause. A dominant lump sometimes forms, requiring a biopsy to confirm the diagnosis. The lump may or may not be painful.

FIBROADENOMAS

Of the fibrocystic changes that develop in women under age 30, half are *fibroadenomas*—very discrete dominant lumps composed of the fibrous tissue and glands adjoining breast ducts. They're generally painless, and a woman may have one or several. They may be round or irregularly shaped, but they can usually be distinctly felt.

Ms. Julie Talbot, age 18, and her mother were very worried when they came to see me after Ms. Talbot had discovered a lump in the upper portion of her left breast. No one in her family had ever had any breast problems, she explained, while I examined what turned out to be a dominant lump one centimeter (a half inch) in diameter. At her age, breast cancer is extremely rare, so the lump was almost certainly a fibroadenoma. It would do her no harm.

I removed the lump because it could present problems. It might grow to a much larger size; it could confuse her doctors as she grew older, and finally, although cancer is extremely rare in an 18-year-old, it can happen. The surgery is a quick outpatient procedure that leaves only a tiny scar, certainly no more unsightly than the lump. The biopsy confirmed it was a fibroadenoma. Ms. Talbot did not even require pain medication. She played tennis a week later.

CYSTOSARCOMA PHYLLOIDES

An unusual tumor, *cystosarcoma phylloides*, occurs mainly in middle-aged women and may grow rapidly to a considerable size—sometimes reaching five centimeters (two inches) in diameter. Despite the cancer-related term *sarcoma* in its name, in the vast majority of situations it is noncancerous. The lump must be removed completely or the portion left behind will continue to grow, giving it some cancer-like characteristics.

MONDOR'S DISEASE

This isn't a disease but an extremely rare change that I've seen only once in my entire practice. It mimics a breast lump, but it's really a line of blood clots that form in the surface veins of the breast. It usually heals without treatment, but a biopsy may be necessary to confirm the diagnosis.

ABSCESS

An *abscess* or boil can form anywhere on the body, including the breasts, when a cut or scrape becomes infected and a pocket of pus forms under the skin. Antibiotics and surgical drainage of the pus generally clear up the problem. Except in nursing mothers, breast abscesses are rare.

MASTITIS

Mastitis may be the most misunderstood fibrocystic change of all, because this term is popularly used (even by some doctors) to describe almost any breast lump or lumpy area. In fact, mastitis is an inflammation or infection in the breast, somewhat like an abscess, that's most common in nursing mothers. If your doctor says you have mastitis, ask if you have a fibrocystic condition and if so, which one, and have him explain that condition to you.

BREAST BUMPS

A lump from a bump? It's rarer than most people think, but you can develop a breast lump from a bump or blow to your breast. The bump ruptures fat cells, other breast cells absorb the fat-cell debris, and a painless lump called *fat necrosis* forms. Because it's a dominant lump, a biopsy is usually needed to make sure of its contents.

Breast bumps and blows do not cause cancer. In my experience, when a woman develops a cancerous lump in a breast that's been bumped, we usually find that the lump has been present for some time but had gone unnoticed. The bump called her attention to it; she hadn't been examining her breasts regularly.

If you consult your doctor about a breast lump or other symptom, chances are she'll be able to reassure you that it is a fibrocystic change. If she does recommend further diagnostic procedures, keep in mind that they are generally quick, inexpensive, and the best means we have for establishing that a breast condition isn't cancerous.

During your breast self-examinations, you will become familiar with any lumps, thickening, or other changes in your breast. If a new lump develops, see your doctor.

6

What Is the Risk of Getting Breast Cancer?

The term *risk factors* is used frequently these days, particularly with regard to breast cancer. From television, newspapers, magazines, and radio come exhortations to eat high-fiber cereal and low-cholesterol foods, to stop smoking, to exercise more—all with the goal of eliminating at least some of the risk that cancer or other diseases will arise.

A risk factor isn't a *cause* of illness, nor does the presence or absence of any risk factor guarantee that illness will or will not occur. It is simply something present more often in people with a disease than in those without that disease.

Doctors suggest that patients take action, if possible, to eliminate or control specific risk factors that may eventually threaten their health. We all know that smokers have a much higher chance of developing lung cancer than nonsmokers. And they *can* stop smoking. But it's not so simple with breast cancer.

We know very little about what actually causes breast cancer or what makes it occur in some women and not in others. We know where it starts and how it spreads (if it does), but we don't know *why*. Nevertheless, some women who get breast cancer blame themselves. Women who are the first in their family to get the disease are especially hard hit by the diagnosis, which seemed so unlikely because they had no genetic predisposition.

It is true that having a family history of breast cancer is associated with a higher risk of getting the disease, but *regardless of risk factors every woman is at risk for developing breast cancer*. About 75 percent of women who do develop breast cancer have no history of the disease in their immediate family and *no* significant risk factors.

Some risk factors—such as having a mother or sister with breast cancer—are not modifiable and are associated more strongly than others with occurrence of the disease. A woman with such "high risk" factors has even greater reason to have her breasts examined frequently. That way, if she does develop breast cancer, it will be discovered early and she'll be in the group for whom treatment is likely to be completely successful.

† The "Bottom Line" Risk of † Developing Breast Cancer

Among all North American women, the risk of getting breast cancer is one in ten. That means that about 100 out of every 1,000 women on this continent will develop breast cancer during their lifetime. If we arbitrarily use a period of fifty years as that portion of a woman's lifetime when she's most vulnerable to breast cancer (from age 30 to age 80), then, of those 1,000 women, on the average about two will get the disease each year.

Older women develop breast cancer at a higher rate than younger women, so actually fewer of the 100 women will get the disease early in life and a larger number will get it later.

These are not particularly useful statistics because there is no way to apply them to an individual woman's concern about getting the disease. And keep in mind that most women who develop breast cancer are found to have no risk factors associated with the disease. This means that *regardless of her risk-factor picture every woman must have regular breast screening for cancer throughout her life after age 30.*

† Major Risk Factor: Family Members † with Breast Cancer

It has been observed over many years that women who have one or more female relatives with breast cancer are more likely to develop the disease themselves. As a result, numerous studies have attempted to determine the risk associated with having a mother, sister, aunt, grandmother, or other female relative with breast cancer. Although researchers have approximately determined the degree of increased risk associated with each of the family patterns, we still have no conclusive information on how or why this happens. It is now believed that several genetic mechanisms may be involved. We have no way to modify this major risk, but we can detect and treat cancer at an early stage if it occurs. (See Table 6-1.)

TABLE 6-1

Assessing Breast Cancer Familial Risk Factors

If there is no family history:	Risk is about 100 out of every 1,000 women
If woman's mother has breast cancer:	Risk is about 170 out of every 1,000 women
If her sister has breast cancer:	Risk is about 150 to 200 out of every 1,000 women
If both her mother and her sister have breast cancer:	Risk is about 200 to 500 out of every 1,000 women
If another family member has breast cancer:	Risk is about 120 to 140 out of every 1,000 women

† MAJOR RISK FACTOR: PREVIOUS †
CANCER IN ONE BREAST

As might be expected, having cancer in one breast increases a woman's risk of developing cancer in the other. This is probably because the two breasts have the same tissue composition and because they are subject to the same hormone and chemical influences in the woman's body. These second-breast cancers appear to be new; that is, they do not seem to have spread from the cancer in the first breast. The risk of a second-breast cancer seems further increased in women who are comparatively young when they first develop the disease.

† Minor Risk Factor: Early †
Onset of Menstruation

Some studies suggest that a girl who begins menstruating before age 12 may have a slightly increased risk of developing breast cancer during her reproductive years; other studies have shown little if any increased risk. Some investigators believe the risk may relate to hormonal changes and imbalances.

† Minor Risk Factor: Late Menopause †

A woman who continues menstruating past age 55 may also have a slightly increased risk of developing breast cancer. Again, this may be due to hormonal influences.

† Minor Risk Factors: Age at †
Time of Pregnancy, Number of Children

A woman who has her first child after age 35, or who has no children, has a slightly increased risk of developing breast cancer. Conversely, a woman who has had her first child before age 20 appears to have a slightly reduced risk, as does a woman who has had several children. Again, hormonal factors are probably involved.

Of course, few women would abandon plans for having children or would have additional children solely on the basis of these minor risk factors.

† Minor Risk Factor: Two Uncommon †
Fibrocystic Changes

Only two comparatively uncommon types of fibrocystic change, atypical ductal hyperplasia and ductal papillomatosis, increase the risk of developing breast cancer. (See page 76.)

† Modifiable Factors That *May* †
or *May Not* Increase Breast Cancer Risk

Post-menopausal use of female hormone medications has been successful in relieving the uncomfortable symptoms of menopause, and women who use them appear to have a lower incidence of cardiovascular disease and osteoporosis. Because hormonal influences also appear to increase or decrease some women's risk of developing breast cancer, these medications have been extensively studied to determine if women who use or have used them in the past are at any increased risk of developing breast cancer.

A 1987 study by the National Cancer Institute and the Center for Disease Control of over 1,300 women with breast cancer failed to show any overall increase in breast cancer in women who had used estrogens.[1] However, a group of over 23,000 women in Sweden were studied and the investigators concluded that there was a very slightly increased risk of developing breast cancer if the medication was taken for more than six years.[2] Yet another study at Harvard University, in which over 33,000 women were investigated, failed to identify any significant increased risk.[3] Each report must be considered in relation to all of the others. Studies will need to investigate tens of thousands of women over several decades to provide definite answers.

If there is any increased risk of developing breast cancer, it is certainly low. It is probably similar to the risk in a woman who has a distant family member with breast cancer. (See page 85.)

However, because we don't have the final answers, women with other risk factors should be concerned when using these medications. If necessary, they should be used for as short a period of time and in as low a dosage as possible.

Birth-control pills (which contain estrogen and progesterone) in use today are not considered a source of increased risk of breast cancer. Because the pill is used by millions of women, a number of research physicians have studied its effects. One hundred and twenty thousand women were questioned by doctors from Harvard Medical School about their use of birth-control pills. No significant increase in the occurrence of breast cancer was noted in women who used the pill for over twenty years.[4]

The Center for Disease Control investigated 4,700 women with newly discovered breast cancer and did not find a greater usage of birth-control pills among these women as compared with a similar group of women without breast cancer.[5] A different type of study at the Roswell Park Memorial Institute failed to show any relation between birth-control pills and breast cancer.[6]

But within such studies some small groups appear to show a *slightly* increased risk of developing breast cancer if a higher-dose birth-control pill was used for a long time. Even though those findings cannot be proven, women are advised to use as low a dosage as is practical. One would certainly expect that if there was a significant risk of breast cancer, some definite trend would have been seen by now, since millions of women take the pill.

† Factors That *Do Not* Increase † Breast Cancer Risk

X-ray dosages used in mammography (see Chapter 3) are very small and *pose no cancer hazard.* X-ray dosages used for treatment after mastectomy and lumpectomy are much larger but do not appear to pose any cancer hazard.

Exposure to some very large X-ray dosages can cause breast cancer. This is what happened to many women (especially very young women and girls) who survived the atom bomb blasts in Hiroshima and Nagasaki in 1945 and women treated years ago with high-dose rays for a variety of conditions. X-rays are no longer used in this manner.

Excessive dietary fat has been thought by some physicians to be a minor risk factor. Women in Asian countries—where meat and fat make up much less of the daily diet than they do in North America and Western Europe—have a much lower incidence of breast cancer. This suggests, but has yet to prove conclusively, that a connection exists.

Therefore, doctors don't yet have the data to recommend limiting dietary fat to prevent breast cancer, but we *do* recommend such a limitation to prevent arteriosclerosis and heart disease. So limiting dietary fat is probably an all-around good idea.

Being overweight, popularly believed to contribute to the development of breast cancer, has not been shown to be a risk factor for the disease. As with limiting dietary fat, avoiding obesity is a generally healthful practice, not a way to prevent breast cancer.

Alcohol. Recent studies at the National Cancer Institute and at Harvard Medical School have shown a slight but measurable increased risk in women who have several drinks per day.[7,8] Reports from the American Health Foundation state that any association of alcohol and breast cancer, if present, is so variable and so weak that no recommendation on its use can be made.[9]

† KEEPING "RISK" IN PERSPECTIVE †

Knowing about risk factors doesn't yet offer a great deal of practical help in the fight against breast cancer. Beyond any consideration of risk factors lies this overriding fact: Only about 25 percent of all women with breast cancer have even one such risk factor. This means that *75 percent of all American women who get breast cancer have no risk factors at all.*

† WHAT ABOUT PREVENTIVE MASTECTOMY? †

The greatest risk of developing breast cancer exists in the rare case when a woman's mother and sister both developed bilateral breast cancer while they were still pre-menopausal. Over the course of a lifetime, such a woman may have up to a fifty-fifty chance of developing breast cancer herself. Women with lobular cancer have a 30 percent or greater chance of having cancer in the opposite breast. Even women with the more common ductal cancer in one breast have an increased risk of developing it in the other breast. These are risks that call for very close and careful screening; in some cases, the woman may want to consider having her breast or breasts surgically removed, with immediate reconstruction (see Chapter 11), before cancer can occur. This operation, *prophylactic* or *preventive mastectomy*, removes the vast majority of the woman's breast tissue. It also removes essentially all of her risk of getting breast cancer, except for cancer that may arise in the very tiny amount of breast tissue remaining under the nipple. To totally prevent cancer, the nipple and areola would also have to be removed.

A controversial form of treatment, it isn't done without the most careful consideration of all the factors involved. But a woman who must otherwise live year in and year out with a high risk of developing breast cancer may elect to have this operation, not only to reduce her risk of getting the disease but also to relieve worry about whether and when it may occur. This operation has been performed at the Mayo Clinic hundreds of times with excellent results. Only 3 women out of over 1,400 high-risk women who had a prophylactic mastectomy at the Clinic have developed cancer in the small amount of remaining breast tissue.[10]

Such excellent results have made this operation more generally accepted. Not every surgeon agrees, but most now feel that if a woman is at high risk and can decrease that risk to almost zero, it is her right to have the operation.

About two years ago I first saw Mrs. Claudia Danz, age 35, for a breast examination and evaluation. She gave me a rather ominous family history. Her mother had died of breast cancer at the age of 40, and her 32-year-old sister recently was discovered to have breast cancer.

I noted no abnormality on breast examination, but a mammogram showed microcalcifications throughout her breasts, with several clustered in one area. This was a very suspicious finding, and the radiologist and I recommended a biopsy of the clustered area. Fortunately, it revealed fibrocystic change, but of a type associated with an increased incidence of breast cancer—atypical ductal hyperplasia.

I explained to her that she had a risk-factor picture that she could not afford to ignore: a very strong family history plus atypical ductal hyperplasia. I could not tell her definitely what her risk of developing breast cancer was, but estimated it could be as high as 30 to 50 percent. At a minimum, I told her, she should have more frequent breast screening than women who are at less risk. I also presented the concept of preventive mastectomy and explained what was involved. I showed her slides of a number of my patients who had had such a mastectomy and reconstruction, including the preservation of the nipple and areola. After this operation, I concluded, she would have almost no chance of developing breast cancer.

She spoke to several other physicians and she returned for a bilateral preventive mastectomy and breast reconstruction. To date, she is doing well.

I now also have a number of young women in my practice who, after having mastectomy and breast reconstruction, have decided to have a preventive mastectomy on the opposite breast. Each was so anxious about the chances of developing a new cancer that after a number of consultations with me and with second-opinion physicians, they decided to have a preventive mastectomy. Of course, I had to warn them that, even with the saving of the nipple and areola, this recon-structed breast would never have the sensation it originally had and would be slightly different in appearance from the other reconstructed breast. And although the risk of devel-oping cancer on that side was very, very low, it still existed since a small amount of breast tissue remains under the nipple. The majority of these women have been pleased with their decision.

7

Breast Cancer:
After the Diagnosis

In the preceding chapters, we've discussed important ways for a woman to care for her breasts. In this and the following chapter, our focus narrows to a discussion of the woman who does get breast cancer and how she and her doctor can work together to plan for the best possible treatment.

This chapter's structure reflects my profound conviction that the "two step" procedure of diagnosing and treating breast cancer is most satisfactory. In this way, the woman decides on her treatment herself. (See Chapter 4.)

† UNDERSTANDING †
BREAST CANCER

When cancer arises anywhere in the body, including the breasts, normal cells (cells that formerly followed orderly structural and growth patterns) change and become cancer cells. We don't know why this change—dramatically apparent under the microscope—occurs, but we do know that it triggers a very aggressive and disorderly growth of the cancer cells. Multiplying, they form into an ever-growing lump. Each such lump has unique characteristics of growth and spread (if any).

Most often, breast cancer arises in the smaller ducts of the breast (ductal cancer). Lobular cancer (arising in the breast lobules or glands) is less common, and cancer ocurring elsewhere in the breast is quite rare. (See Diagram 7-1.)

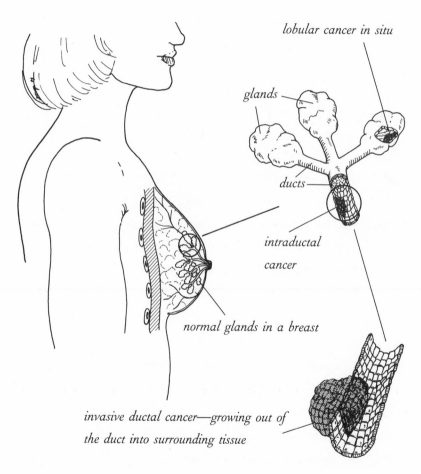

lobular cancer in situ

glands

ducts

intraductal cancer

normal glands in a breast

invasive ductal cancer—growing out of the duct into surrounding tissue

DIAGRAM 7-1   Where Common Types of
Breast Cancers Develop

Although cancerous tissue generally grows faster than normal tissue, most breast cancers appear to have been present and growing for three to five years before they can be seen on a mammogram and for five to seven years before they are large enough to be felt.

Recently a patient referred her 33-year-old daughter, Mrs. Anne Johnson, to me for a routine breast examination and mammogram. When the daughter requested that the mammogram be performed at a place other than where her mother's had been taken, I asked why, expecting her to tell me that the examination was very painful. Instead, she said, "You told my mother that her cancer had been growing for five years, and since she had had a number of previous mammograms, obviously it was missed." Surprised, I explained that although the cancer had been growing for a long time, *it was undetectable by any means then or now available to us.*

† CANCER GROWTH PATTERNS †

We now know that the growth of cancer isn't the orderly process it was formerly believed to be. For example, the lymph nodes in the armpit aren't always the first target of cancer invasion beyond the breast tissues; breast cancer can spread at any time to any part of the body without invading the lymph nodes first.

Cancer cells do not usually enter the lymphatics or blood vessels when they first develop. But as their growth continues, the cells of some—not all—cancers may spread into the lymphatics or blood vessels, traveling to the lymph nodes and to distant body areas such as the bones, lungs, or liver. This is known as *metastasis*. Even when cancer cells escape the original cancer site, they don't always start growing in the areas to which they travel, or they may form in some areas they reach but not in others.

But although cancer spread is very unpredictable, we *do* *know* that there is a connection between the presence of cancer cells in the underarm lymph nodes and the likelihood that, eventually, cancer will arise elsewhere in the woman's body. This is why it is usually necessary to remove those lymph nodes to see if they do contain cancer. If they do, then the woman is at a higher risk of further spread. The oncologist and surgeon use this information in determining the woman's need for adjuvant therapy to lessen the likelihood of metastases.

† CLASSIFICATION AND STAGING †

Before doctor and patient can decide on specific treatment options, they need to know the degree to which the cancer involves the patient's body, and they need to know the cancer's characteristics. *Classification* describes the particular type of cancer that is present. *Staging* describes its growth in terms of physical characteristics: invasive or noninvasive, size, lymph node involvement, and spread to distant areas of the body.

† "THE DIAGNOSIS IS CANCER" †

It is always difficult for a woman and her doctor to discuss the fact that her breast biopsy results show cancer.

†

Mrs. Nancy Louis, age 42, had a breast biopsy and was found to have a one-centimeter (one-half-inch) invasive ductal cancer in her right breast. As soon as I walked into the examining room where she had been sent to have her biopsy dressing changed, I told her that we had found a small but very treatable breast cancer. This news is always such a shock that considerably more discussion is needed before the woman is able to face her condition, understand it, and make rational decisions about her treatment. I explained that I would change her dressing and then sit down with her in my office (along with anyone she wanted with her for support) to discuss the entire situation.

Understandably, she was upset, so I allowed enough time for her to compose herself somewhat. Then, after she was dressed, our nurse brought her and her husband into my office, where we spent the next forty-five minutes discussing her particular cancer. We also spoke at length about the various types and combinations of treatment that had the best chance of eradicating it. By the time she left my office, she had achieved some measure of control over her fear, and she was concentrating on making the necessary decisions about her treatment. Although a long road lay ahead, she had taken the first courageous step.

† Talking with Your Doctor †

Of course, no two doctors are alike, and every patient-doctor relationship is unique. But any woman with breast cancer should expect her doctor to:

- tell her first that she has the disease and explain her condition clearly

- describe her particular type of breast cancer to the best of his ability
- be aware of and discuss all the suitable treatment options
- discuss her disease, treatment, and prognosis only with her and family members or friends she designates, if any
- answer all her questions frankly and fully
- suggest consultation with other doctors, such as an oncologist or another surgeon, and keep her informed about their opinions and recommendations
- allow her to select the treatment(s) she'll receive
- respond sensitively to her statements and questions about her chances for successful treatment, always holding out hope that she will be in the group that have no further problems
- avoid communicating anxiety or discomfort about her disease
- provide support for her and suggest other sources of aid, such as groups for women with breast cancer
- assure her that, as the years pass, he will continue to follow her progress, performing regular checkups and remaining available to answer her questions and help with problems that might develop
- be a source of new information concerning breast cancer as it becomes available

† CLASSIFICATION OF NONINVASIVE † BREAST CANCER

As I've noted above, whether cancer arises in a breast duct (ductal) or gland (lobular), it's considered noninvasive if biopsy shows it hasn't spread out of the duct or lobule to invade the surrounding breast structures.

Intraductal cancer is cancer that hasn't spread from its original site in a breast duct. On the whole, it has the highest rate of successful treatment—approaching 100 percent. If intraductal cancer isn't treated, or if treatment is delayed, eventually the cancer cells spread from the original site inside the duct to become invasive. This cancer occurs in basically two forms: most commonly a single small lump or occasionally in multiple ducts throughout a larger portion of the breast.

Lobular cancer in situ is noninvasive cancer arising in a breast lobule. Little is understood about this form of noninvasive cancer and what is known is confusing. Although less common than intraductal cancer, it is more problematic. Most often occurring in younger women, these cancers don't usually form lumps that can be felt or seen on mammography, so they are typically discovered only when a woman's breast is biopsied for another reason.

Studies have shown that women with lobular cancer in situ frequently develop invasive cancer in the same breast, the opposite breast, or both breasts. These invasive cancers don't appear to be extensions of the lobular cancer in situ; rather, they are new cancers. Many of these new cancers are not even lobular cancers. Therefore most specialists consider this type of noninvasive cancer to be a risk factor for invasive cancer rather than a definite cancer itself. Still others believe it is already an early form of breast cancer. This confusion is further compounded when one has to decide upon treatment.

† Classification of Invasive † Breast Cancer

Some 85 to 90 percent of all breast cancers are classified as *invasive ductal cancer*. Probably starting out as intraductal cancer, this cancer, which may arise in several ducts simultaneously, eventually grows through the duct walls and invades surrounding breast tissues. Frequently we see intraductal cancer and invasive ductal cancer in the same area. It is usually confined to one breast, although the opposite breast is at a higher risk for developing cancer in the future than the breasts of women without breast cancer.

Invasive lobular cancer accounts for less than 10 percent of breast cancers. About one third of women with this type of cancer will eventually develop a new cancer in the opposite breast.

Inflammatory breast cancer, also an invasive ductal cancer, occurs infrequently—about 1 percent of all breast cancers—but is much more aggressive. Cancer cells fill the skin's lymphatic ducts until the skin over the breast becomes red and painful, mimicking an infection. Because this type of cancer grows so rapidly, the long-term outlook is not good, although with newer methods of treatment it is improving.

Other types of breast cancer originate from other cells in the breast, such as muscle and blood vessels. These are so rare that should a biopsy diagnose such a cancer, treatment must be considered on an individual basis. Even though they originate in the breast, they are not typical breast cancers.

† STAGING BREAST CANCER †

· What should initial treatment be for a woman diagnosed as having breast cancer?

· Will she need adjuvant treatment with chemotherapy, irradiation, or hormonal therapy afterward?

The answers to these questions depend on accurate cancer staging as well as classification. Staging occurs in two phases: before and after the initial treatment. *Clinical staging* is based on clinical examination and biopsy findings. Although it provides important guidelines for treatment planning, it is not as accurate as post-treatment *pathological staging*—examination of all the surgically removed tissue. The final decisions regarding adjuvant treatment depend upon it. This has been proven a number of times, such as recently in an ongoing study by the National Cancer Institute of almost 25,000 women with breast cancer. The size of the cancer and the involvement of the lymph nodes were the two most important indicators of a woman's chances for successful recovery from cancer.[1]

Surgical removal of the underarm lymph nodes for microscopic analysis is the *only* way to learn whether they contain cancer and, if so, to what extent. A doctor would be incorrect in his diagnosis far too often if he relied solely on feeling beneath the arm to determine if cancerous lymph nodes were present.

Doctors most commonly use the so-called TNM system— for *T*umor (sizes), *N*ode (extent of lymph node involvement, if any), and *M*etastases (presence, if any, of distant metastases)—to stage breast cancer. Each stage in this system

(I–IV, with several substage categories) takes into account all three of these factors. A commission of several large national organizations have developed the consensus classification.[2]

The TNM Cancer Staging System

Stage	Size	Lymph Node Involvement	Spread to Distant Sites
0 (noninvasive)	Any Size	No	No
I	2 cm or less	No	No
IIa	2 cm or less	Yes	No
	2 to 5 cm	No	No
IIb	2 to 5 cm	Yes	No
	over 5 cm	No	No
IIIa	5 cm or less	Yes (extensive)	No
	over 5 cm	Any	No
IIIb	Extensive	Yes (extensive)	No
IV	Any size	Yes or No	Yes

† Deciding on Breast Cancer Treatment †

Until about thirty years ago, there was only one treatment for breast cancer: extensive surgical removal of the breast and surrounding tissues by the now obsolete operation known as the Halsted radical mastectomy. There were no decisions to be made; immediately after analysis of the biopsy indicated that cancer was present, a radical mastectomy was performed.

Today, a number of treatments are available for the woman with breast cancer. That's why the "two step" procedure of biopsy and a waiting period followed by surgery is most often used (and should be used in almost every situation). One or two days after the biopsy, the woman and her doctor discuss the classification, the clinical staging, and the treatment options available, along with her recommendation for treatment. The patient also is able to discuss these matters with her family and obtain another doctor's opinion before she makes the final treatment decision.

Many decisions must be made after I explain the diagnosis to my patient. But I emphasize that she need not make all these decisions right away. She needs to decide on what initial, or primary, treatment she will have (assuming that in her particular situation she has a choice of two or more treatment options).

Adjuvant treatment—chemotherapy, irradiation therapy, or hormonal therapy, begun several weeks after the initial treatment is finished—will almost always be recommended. However, decisions about adjuvant treatment are not usually made until pathological staging is complete, unless the cancer requires pre-treatment with chemotherapy and/or irradiation. Most often, the woman and her treatment team will take time to study the pathological reports and decide together on the best adjuvant treatment for her.

† Understanding †
Clinical Studies

Studies using actual patients are the last stage in a long process of testing new treatment methods. At this point, the goal of the studies is to compare the new methods with each other and with older treatments to learn which are most effective—or are equally effective with the advantage of causing less physical trauma for the patient.

Because the word "study" implies experimentation, some women may fear that they would receive inadequate treatment in a study. No woman participating in any segment of a well-thought-out study will be treated by a method that is known to be inadequate.

For over fifty years after Dr. William S. Halsted described and popularized the radical mastectomy, no other treatments were even seriously considered. In its day, the radical mastectomy certainly saved lives, but at the cost of massive chest deformity and psychological trauma for the women involved. If no clinical studies had been done to develop equally effective and less traumatic methods of treatment, the Halsted procedure would still be our treatment of choice today.

One of the first nationwide studies, the National Surgical Adjuvant Breast and Bowel Project (NSABP), accumulated data from over twenty-five large institutions in the United States to study many facets in the treatment of breast cancer. One of their first projects attempted to prove whether a lesser type of mastectomy was as good as Halsted's radical mastectomy. They randomly assigned women with breast cancer to have either a radical mastectomy or the new and not yet fully accepted modified radical mastectomy. The study proved that both operations were equally effective.[3]

Later, other studies showed that the breast-conservation procedures appeared to be as effective in many women as the modified radical mastectomy—while saving the breast. Studies have also proven that chemotherapy and hormonal therapy are very effective.

† Present and †
Future Benefits

You may be wondering why thousands of women would agree to treatment in clinical trials when continued treatment by their own doctors alone might be more comfortable and reassuring.

Doctors, and increasing numbers of people in our society, recognize the enormous contributions such studies make to our understanding of breast cancer treatment. Thus, a woman taking part in such a study is contributing not only to her own recovery but also to the recovery of thousands of women who in the future will benefit from treatment based on the study results.

† Two Study Methods †

Clinical studies must be structured and implemented scientifically. That can be difficult when researchers are dealing with a disease as complex as breast cancer, but it's the only way to obtain information that can later be applied to patients outside the study. In general, there are two basic approaches to studying breast cancer treatment: retrospective studies and prospective studies (clinical trials). Retrospective studies— studies of groups of women whose treatment has already been started or even completed—have previously been the most widely used. But clinical trials, which are carefully planned *before* any treatment begins, can provide much more reliable information.

† WHAT HAPPENS †
IN A CLINICAL TRIAL?

A clinical trial for breast cancer treatment requires large numbers of women (hundreds or even thousands) whose treatment can be modified to try to improve the present treatment. To put together such a large study, physicians from several hospitals and medical centers frequently arrange to pool the information they gather.

To begin a clinical trial, women with similar breast cancers (and other characteristics, such as age) are divided into two or more groups, and each woman is randomly placed into one of the groups. One group might be treated in the traditional way using surgery without adjuvant therapy, and the other group might be treated with the addition of adjuvant therapy. Then the investigators regularly evaluate the treatment results, monitoring how each group does over the years.

If the group of women who received adjuvant as well as traditional surgical therapy had better results than those women who received only the traditional therapy, then a benefit from the addition of adjuvant therapy is considered to have been proved, and the new treatment can be provided for women outside the study. Although studies may continue for years, investigators can use sophisticated statistical analysis to come up with early indications of treatment outcomes. So the benefits of improved treatment can become clear fairly early in a study, after just a few years.

Of course, enrolling for treatment in a prospective clinical trial is a big step for a woman. The doctor always explains that certain treatment options apply in her case. He may then recommend that his patient consider entering a clinical study that would not jeopardize her chances for a successful treatment outcome no matter which group she was placed in. A National Institute of Health Consensus strongly recommends participation in clinical studies as the only way to develop the best treatment methods.

Prior to entering a study, the patient must have the following information:

- how the particular study the doctor is recommending corresponds with the generally accepted methods of breast cancer treatment
- why, if the study includes taking drugs, she may not be told what drug she is taking
- what her rights and obligations are as a study participant,

including her right to withdraw from the study at any time and her obligation to accept treatment by a different doctor, usually the one coordinating the study

- the fact that she will need to sign a form called "informed consent," indicating that she has received a full explanation of the study.

8

Basic Information for the Treatment of Breast Cancer

As seen in the preceding chapter, initial and adjuvant breast cancer treatment is based largely on the classification and staging of the cancer—its type, size, degree of spread beyond the original site, and the receptor status.

Three general areas must be considered in planning treatment for breast cancer: the breast itself, where *local* treatment is applied to minimize the chance that the cancer will recur in that breast; the lymph nodes under the arms, or *regional* area, which are analyzed after surgical removal to provide information on prognosis; and the woman's need for *systemic* treatment (hormonal therapy or chemotherapy) for her entire body.

Whatever treatment plan a woman and her doctors select, the first goal is complete removal of the cancer known to be present, the second goal is to minimize the chance of cancer regrowth (recurrence) in the breast, and the third goal is to minimize the chance of cancer occurring elsewhere. These goals must be accomplished with as little traumatic effect on the woman's body as possible.

Before she reaches a final decision, a woman with breast

cancer should consider *all* the possible treatments that could be appropriate for her individual condition. Dealing with all of this information can be trying and confusing, especially at a time when she and her family are upset and worried and especially if, as sometimes happens, different doctors make different treatment recommendations. This chapter will help a woman in this difficult situation keep the facts straight and understand her condition fully in her discussions with her doctor, the surgeon, the oncologist, and any other doctor or caregiver she consults.

† Primary Local and Regional † Treatments Used Today

Modified Radical Mastectomy

By the 1950s, doctors were beginning to note a trend toward detection of breast cancer at earlier stages than was formerly the case. With these smaller cancers, only rarely were extensive amounts of skin or the muscles beneath the breast affected. This seemed to suggest that the Halsted radical mastectomy could be *modified* to remove only the breast, a small amount of skin, and the lymph nodes in the armpit, leaving the chest-wall muscles and most of the skin intact. (Diagrams 8-1 and 8-1A.) Surgeons started performing this less deforming mastectomy and then clinical studies proved its effectiveness.

The deformity caused by a modified radical mastectomy is still significant. The skin lies directly on the pectoralis muscle

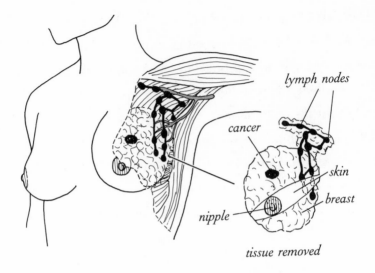

DIAGRAM 8-1   Modified Radical Mastectomy

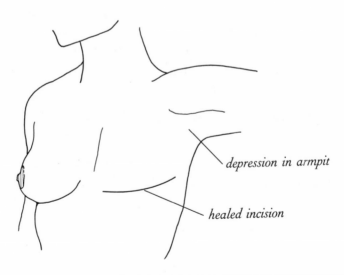

DIAGRAM 8-1A   Appearance After Modified Radical Mastectomy

and no breast mound is present. A depression in the armpit is left where the lymph nodes were removed. However, by leaving the breast muscle (pectoralis) in place and minimizing loss of chest skin, it makes breast reconstruction much simpler.

The modified radical mastectomy has become the standard for breast cancer surgery, but in many cases an even simpler procedure, breast conservation, may also be used. (See page 114.)

SIMPLE (TOTAL) MASTECTOMY

The simple or total mastectomy is similar to the modified radical mastectomy except that the armpit lymph nodes are *not* removed. A few lymph nodes in the area where the breast joins the lymph node tissue are incidentally taken out with the breast.

Treatment by simple mastectomy may be indicated in the following circumstances:

- when the woman has intraductal (noninvasive) breast cancer. There is such a low likelihood of spread to the armpit lymph nodes that I and most surgeons do not remove them.
- when the woman is very ill and it is desirable to perform only the simplest operation. This operation takes less than half as long to perform as a modified radical mastectomy.
- when removal of lymph nodes for staging isn't necessary because the woman's cancer is known to have spread elsewhere in the body. The simple mastectomy is done

to provide some measure of local control of cancer where complete eradication is no longer an option.

BREAST-CONSERVATION THERAPY: LUMPECTOMY, REMOVAL OF AX-ILLARY LYMPH NODES, AND IRRADIATION

When a woman's breast cancer is small or moderate-sized, the doctor should offer an alternative to modified radical mastectomy: a breast-conservation technique using the *combination* treatment of:

1. lumpectomy, plus
2. lymph node removal for staging purposes, followed by
3. irradiation of the remaining breast tissue over a period of four to six weeks.

With this three-part procedure, the breast is saved. (Diagrams 8-2 and 8-2A.) If her surgeon cannot recommend breast conservation, he should at least explain to her why not. This form of treatment is increasingly chosen by women who have the option.

A *lumpectomy* involves the removal of the cancer and a small amount of surrounding breast tissue. In most cases, like mastectomy, lumpectomy is performed as the second step of the two-step biopsy/surgery procedure and at the same time as the underarm lymph nodes are removed. Sometimes the lumpectomy portion of the treatment may be performed during the biopsy procedure if the surgeon can remove a small amount of normal breast tissue around the cancer without causing a deformity. If cancer is diagnosed, the surgeon will only have

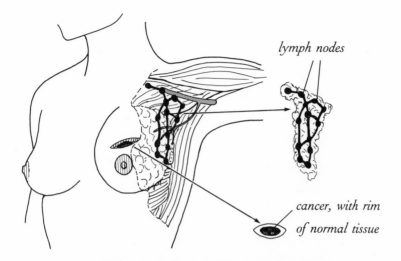

lymph nodes

*cancer, with rim
of normal tissue*

DIAGRAM 8-2   Breast-Conservation Surgery:
Lumpectomy and Removal of Lymph Nodes

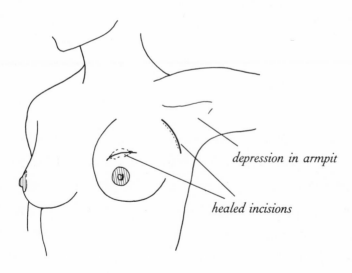

depression in armpit

healed incisions

DIAGRAM 8-2A   Appearance After Breast Conservation

to perform the staging lymph node removal at a later date.

We have about twenty years' worth of study data proving the effectiveness of breast conservation. A large study from France has shown no difference in the outcome of 300 women treated with breast conservation as opposed to mastectomy.[1] At the M. D. Anderson Hospital in Dallas, Texas, over 1,000 women treated by one of the two methods demonstrated no difference in recurrence rates.[2] Similar results were found in a smaller study from Los Angeles.[3]

A very impressive prospective study from Milan, Italy, involving 700 women confirmed that a radical mastectomy had no advantage over breast conservation.[4] In the largest, most complete prospective project ever undertaken, the National Surgical Adjuvant Breast and Bowel Project (NSABP) has followed over 2,000 women at about twenty-five hospitals for at least five to ten years (many longer) and demonstrated that breast conservation is as effective as mastectomy.[5,6] My and most other breast cancer specialists' expectation is that future studies will confirm this finding for even longer periods of time.

As much as we might wish it, lumpectomy isn't always a good choice for breast cancer treatment even when a woman's cancer is small. If a cancer is located just below the nipple or areola, the lumpectomy would necessitate removing the nipple and areola plus surrounding tissue from the center of the breast, markedly deforming it. In that case, the surgeon may recommend a modified radical mastectomy with immediate reconstruction. But if the woman can accept the added deformity in the center of her breast, breast conservation is still possible.

Lumpectomy is also *inadvisable*:

* when the same breast has two or more cancers not close together
* in some cases when there is cancer in both breasts
* when the cancer is large in proportion to the size of the breast
* when the cancer cannot be completely removed without markedly deforming the breast
* when intraductal cancer extends out into other areas of the breast from the principal cancer

For maximum effectiveness, lumpectomy is always combined with irradiation treatment of the remaining breast tissue. Studies show a high likelihood (over 30 percent) of recurring cancer in the breast after lumpectomy *if no irradiation is given*.[5] That is not acceptable treatment. With a full course of adjuvant irradiation therapy, however, breast conservation has essentially the *same* five- to ten-year low local recurrence rate as modified radical mastectomy.

The NSABP studies have also shown that, should the cancer recur in the breast after lumpectomy and irradiation, most of the affected women can then be successfully treated by mastectomy.

Because irradiation therapy involves many different considerations, each woman's treatment must be tailored specifically for her. Usually she will receive daily treatment over a four- to six-week period, five days per week, at a hospital or medical center near her home. Irradiation dosage is measured in rads; for breast cancer, a typical cancer-killing dose is about 5,000 to 6,000 rads (also called centi-Grays). That's the *total* dose, commonly administered at around 180 to 200 rads per day over the treatment period.

The exact area where the cancer arose in the breast is frequently given a somewhat higher dosage, called a *boost*. Amounting to about 1,000 additional rads, it may be given either in the usual way or by insertion of radioactive needles into the cancer area.

After breast irradiation, the unavoidable injury to some normal cells typically causes slight thickening of the skin and underlying breast tissue. The breast usually becomes slightly firmer due to skin shrinkage, and the skin may temporarily redden, peel, and/or "weep" and become more sensitive. Other mild side effects include nausea and/or temporary difficulty in swallowing. Slight scarring of the underlying lung can also occur but almost never causes harm. Only rarely does the therapy reduce the body's ability to produce white blood cells; when this happens, the treatments may need to be spaced further apart.

How safe is irradiation? Most of the data we have now indicate that it causes only minimal damage to normal breast tissue and is quite safe. We don't know definitely that today's irradiation doses *never* cause any new cancer to develop, but we have certainly not seen any evidence of it.

Of course, women with breast cancer who are in their 30s, 40s, and 50s are concerned with surviving quite a bit longer than five or ten years—more like forty years. Frankly, we don't yet have the data on how the outcomes of lumpectomy will compare with the outcomes of modified radical mastectomy after that many years. Lumpectomy is still too new for the necessary studies, now underway, to have been completed. *But every indication is that lumpectomy will be as good a treatment as mastectomy even over the long term.* Today, women who are considering lumpectomy/breast conservation for breast cancer treatment must understand that the long-term outcome of their decision, although predictably as good as the outcome would be for modified radical mastectomy, is not yet completely supported by study results.

BREAST IRRADIATION TREATMENT

Very occasionally, irradiation treatment is selected as the sole primary therapy by women who refuse surgery or who cannot tolerate it for health reasons.

Treatment of any cancer with irradiation (X-rays) is based on the medical principle that hitting living cancer cells with a beam from an X-ray tube will kill them. Fortunately, destroying cancer cells this way usually requires less irradiation than is needed to destroy normal cells. The radiotherapist selects the dosage that will do maximum damage to cancer cells with minimal damage to normal ones.

† ADJUVANT OR ADDITIONAL TREATMENTS †

Adjuvant therapies are treatments given in addition to and usually after the primary treatment, to lessen the chances of cancer recurring in the breast area itself or elsewhere in the body.

Adjuvant Irradiation Therapy

The efficacy of irradiation as primary treatment of breast cancer has been proven in the breast conservation studies. But it has also been shown to be effective as an adjuvant therapy after mastectomy for women with large breast cancers. It reduces the chances of local cancer recurrence in the breast area, especially if the cancer was near the edge of the breast tissue removed. I strongly suggest consultation with a radiotherapist for any woman with such a cancer.

As far back as the 1920s, women were treated with irradiation after undergoing mastectomies. Initially, studies showed no clear-cut improvement in overall survival rates for these women, so the value of adjuvant irradiation therapy remained unproven until recently. Radiotherapists speculate that the earlier failure of irradiation therapy to improve overall survival rates may have been attributable to less than adequate doses.

Irradiation can even be used with women who have undergone immediate reconstruction. It usually causes some firmness or even slight deformity of the reconstructed breast, but these complications are relatively minor or can be corrected.

Irradiation therapy is *not* used as adjuvant therapy for women whose only indication of cancer spread is involvement of regional lymph nodes. These women are treated with hormonal therapy or chemotherapy.

† Adjuvant Systemic Treatments †

Because breast cancer can spread beyond the breast and the lymph nodes under the arm to start new cancers in distant areas of the body—the process known as *metastasis*—systemic treatment (treatment that affects the entire body) is frequently recommended. It is never known if these metastases will occur, so the goal of such adjuvant therapy is to lessen the likelihood.

Chemotherapy and hormonal therapy, the two main types of systemic treatments, decrease the likelihood of metastases in many women.

Systemic therapy is a complex specialty in itself. It is usually administered and managed by an oncologist in cooperation with the woman's surgeon. Most of my patients with breast cancer consult with oncologists, at my recommendation, and I strongly urge such consultation for most women with breast cancer.

Systemic therapy is referred to as *adjuvant therapy* if we don't know whether cancer spread has occurred or not. It is known as *treatment of advanced breast cancer* if the cancer is known to have spread beyond the breast or lymph nodes—for example, to the bones or lung. For such advanced cancer, systemic therapy is the principal treatment. When only a single metastatic lesion is found, irradiation therapy may also be used.

Our striving for the most effective and least toxic regimen has led to the development of numerous types of systemic therapy. New recommendations appear monthly in medical publications, making consultation with an oncologist imperative.

† Hormonal Therapy †

In the late nineteenth century, doctors discovered that removing the ovaries of women with breast cancer—the sources of the female hormone estrogen—sometimes slowed or stopped the progress of the disease. We now know that estrogen stimulates the growth of many breast cancer cells. For many years, surgery to remove the ovaries or irradiation to stop their functioning was the only "hormonal treatment" available.

Today, doctors frequently use the anti-estrogen drug tamoxifen (Nolvadex) to slow cancer cell growth by blocking the cancer-stimulating effect of estrogen. Because of the availability and effectiveness of this drug, ovary removal or irradiation is rarely necessary today. Hormonal therapy is *only* effective in women who have high estrogen receptor levels in their cancer.

In the 1960s and 1970s, chemicals called *estrogen receptors* and *progesterone receptors* were identified in some women's breast cancer cells. Investigators found that when present in the cancer cell, these chemicals attract circulating estrogen or progesterone, combine with it, and somehow increase the growth of the cancer. Paradoxically, they also discovered that when these receptors were present in sufficient amounts, the chances for successful treatment seemed better. We can easily test for the presence of these receptor cells in women with breast cancer (it should always be done), and that information is included in formulating the woman's treatment. We understand much less about the purposes of progesterone receptors.

Sometimes a cancer is too tiny to be analyzed, but the woman may still receive hormonal treatment in the hope that high estrogen receptor levels were present, especially if she is post-menopausal. Hormonal treatment generally causes less discomfort and fewer side effects than chemotherapy. But its action against cancer cells is slow compared with chemotherapy's more immediate effects. Hormonal therapy alone is sometimes recommended by oncologists for women who have involvement of none or only a few lymph nodes.

A 1989 NSABP report shows that even if no lymph nodes are involved, fewer women (with estrogen receptors) have recurrence of their cancer when given hormonal therapy.[7] The improvement was slight because these women already do quite well even without adjuvant therapy. During the study 83 percent remained disease-free if they took tamoxifen, compared with 77 percent without tamoxifen. With these outstanding results, the researchers decided to discontinue the clinical trial so everyone could be offered hormonal therapy if they had estrogen receptors present.

Tamoxifen, the drug most frequently used for hormonal therapy, is taken orally, twice a day, and can cost over $50 per month. The side effects are minimal, but in premenopausal women hormonal therapy usually causes premature onset of menopause. It is taken for a minimum of five years and maybe for a lifetime.

† CHEMOTHERAPY †

The use of chemical agents as systemic therapy for breast cancer began in the 1950s, when several types of drugs were developed that destroyed cancer cells or prevented their growth. First used in women with advanced breast cancer, they soon proved their additional worth as adjuvant therapy, significantly lengthening the period of disease-free and overall survival in an NSABP study. The improvement was 5 to 8 percent using rather primitive regimens of chemotherapy.[8]

The effectiveness of chemotherapy does not depend on estrogen receptors being present. There's no doubt that adjuvant chemotherapy improves the odds against breast cancer recurrence. Women with high levels of estrogen receptors may receive *both* hormonal therapy and chemotherapy.

Today, chemotherapy is recommended for adjuvant therapy for women with cancerous lymph node involvement. But recent studies from the NSABP,[9] Europe,[10] and the Eastern Cooperative Oncology Group[11] show that women with no cancer in their lymph nodes may also benefit from chemotherapy if they do not have estrogen receptors.

† CHEMOTHERAPY DRUGS AND † HOW THEY WORK

There are various categories of chemotherapy drugs, but all of them have as their goal maximum destruction of cancer cells with minimal damage to normal ones. The drugs circulate throughout the body, affecting all the tissues; most frequently combinations of several different chemotherapy drugs are used at the same time.

Chemotherapy drugs work on cells that are growing rapidly—and cancer cells grow or multiply faster than the normal cells. The drugs' effect on normal cells is what causes the side effects commonly associated with chemotherapy. It is important for the woman to understand how and why these changes occur.[12]

METHODS OF ADMINISTRATION

There are essentially three methods of administering chemotherapeutic agents. There is no choice of which method to use for a particular drug; rather, the characteristics of the drug dictate which to use:

Intravenous or IV. Injection directly into the bloodstream is especially useful for rapid drug absorption and for drugs that are very irritating when injected into a muscle. The blood provides immediate dilution, reducing the drugs' potential for irritation.

Intramuscular or IM. Injection into a muscle, usually in the buttocks but sometimes in the arm, is generally done when the doctor wants to avoid too rapid absorption of particularly strong drugs.

Oral. The drugs are absorbed by the stomach or intestinal lining before they take effect. This method works well if the drugs do not injure the stomach walls and if they can be absorbed by the cells of the stomach or intestinal lining.

The treatments may be given in the hospital (if the woman is hospitalized) or in the patient's home, but they are most often given in a clinic or doctor's office. The length of time over which chemotherapy needs to be administered varies greatly, from three months to as long as two years, averaging six to twelve months.

FREQUENCY OF TREATMENTS

Oral chemotherapeutic agents are usually administered daily or for a number of days in a row. IV or IM injection schedules can vary widely, from daily administration over several days (followed by a period of rest before the next treatment) to single administrations given at three- or four-week intervals.

UNDERSTANDING CHEMOTHERAPY SIDE EFFECTS

Chemotherapeutic drugs affect normal body tissues—most often the bone marrow, hair follicles, gastrointestinal tract (including the mouth), skin, and sexual organs, causing uncomfortable or undesirable side effects. Taking these strong drugs also causes fatigue and, sometimes, weight gain.

Bone marrow. Most chemotherapeutic drugs destroy some of the bone marrow cells that manufacture red and white blood cells, platelets, and other blood products. The *white blood cells* (WBCs) normally fight infections that the body is exposed to. When WBCs are decreased during chemotherapy, the woman's infection-fighting ability will be reduced until her bone marrow is again able to produce the normal number of WBCs—usually several weeks after chemotherapy.

During this period the doctor will monitor her WBC count carefully, measuring it by means of a simple blood test. (This test will also be done just before the next treatment, to ensure that her WBC count has returned to a safe level.) She must take extra care to avoid infection, and she should notify her doctor at the first sign that she has one.

Chemotherapy also reduces the number of *red blood cells* (RBCs); the resulting anemia may cause extreme fatigue. Reduced numbers of *platelets* can make the woman more susceptible to bruising and bleeding.

Fortunately these problems do not generally persist once the woman's chemotherapy has been completed.

Hair follicles. The hair follicles (cells beneath the scalp that produce the hair shafts) are very active; consequently, they are very sensitive to injury such as that caused by chemotherapeutic drugs. When the follicles are injured, they produce brittle hair that easily breaks off at the scalp. The amount of hair loss during chemotherapy can range from only a slight thinning to complete baldness, but this is almost always only a temporary condition.

Sometimes—with the oncologist's approval—a cold cap can be worn during the treatment, to reduce the amount of blood flowing to the scalp, minimizing the drugs' contact with hair follicles.

Gastrointestinal tract. The gastrointestinal (GI) tract is severely affected by chemotherapeutic drugs, which can cause mouth soreness and dryness, nausea, vomiting, and diarrhea. Mouth soreness can be avoided or minimized by not eating acid or salty foods, by using a soft toothbrush, and by rinsing the mouth frequently. The severity of nausea, vomiting, and diarrhea varies from drug to drug and from woman to woman. Fortunately, today's anti-nausea medications can be effective in controlling nausea and vomiting, particularly if the woman also eats small, light meals during the treatment, drinks little liquid while eating, and rests afterward. The doctor can prescribe medications for diarrhea if it occurs.

Skin. Skin redness, itching, peeling, and dryness are common side effects of the various chemotherapeutic drugs. Frequent applications of skin lotion can help relieve these irritations, and prescription medications are available if needed.

Sexual organs. Many chemotherapeutic drugs will cause menstruation to stop, either temporarily or permanently. They can also cause temporary or even permanent infertility. Other effects of the drugs on sexual organs include vaginal dryness, "hot flashes," and decreased sexual desire, all usually temporary.

Fatigue. While receiving chemotherapy, many women tire easily and need more rest than usual. This results partly from the development of anemia to the drugs' effect on the red blood cells. But most often, fatigue probably stems from the generally powerful effect of these strong drugs on the woman's body. Getting plenty of rest, avoiding stress, eating well, and generally taking good care of herself are a woman's best choices for minimizing fatigue during chemotherapy.

Weight gain. Although not completely understood, weight gain during chemotherapy is thought to occur in part because of decreased metabolism, lessened physical activity, and a tendency to retain fluids in the body. It is usually a temporary situation, although it is sometimes difficult to lose the weight after the therapy has been concluded.

9

Specific Treatment Recommendations for Breast Cancer

Deciding on treatment for breast cancer is surely one of the most complex and emotionally charged situations a woman can face. Yet the vast majority of the women I see display remarkable courage as well as sound thinking at this very stressful time in their lives.

When I tell a woman that she has breast cancer, both of us are uncomfortable at first. I don't like to be the bearer of such upsetting news, and she doesn't like receiving it. Immediately after hearing the diagnosis, the woman is likely to find it difficult to absorb any information besides the single enormous fact of having breast cancer. To help her get by this impasse and begin to understand her situation, I try to give her as much information as I can. That way, my patient bases her decisions on the clearest possible picture of the facts of her case.

Gradually, she finds the strength to listen and relisten to the treatment options available for her type and stage of cancer and to ask questions that will help her decide among them.

Before her treatment is selected (and sometimes at intervals after it's completed), a woman may undergo one or more tests designed to make her specific cancer picture as clear as possible.

Chest X-ray. Every woman with breast cancer should have an initial chest X-ray examination and should also have one at least once a year. It is very unusual to find metastatic cancer in the lungs when breast cancer is first discovered, but the initial examination provides a baseline for future chest X-rays.

Bone scan. After intravenous injection of radioisotopes, which accumulate in large amounts in areas of abnormal bone growth, X-ray examination of the body's entire bone structure reveals any such areas, which may or may not be cancerous. (Abnormal bone conditions such as arthritis or healed fractures are much more common than cancer.) With early-stage cancer, less than 3 to 7 percent of women will have cancer spread to bone, whereas in later stages, the figure rises to 25 percent.

Liver scan. Radiologists also use radioisotopes and X-ray examination to detect abnormal growths in the liver. Because the liver is not initially involved in the spread of cancer, this test is rarely done except in later-stage breast cancer.

CT (computerized tomography) scan. A CT scan is a special X-ray of the body that can examine specific organ tissues, such as the liver, and detect the presence of metastatic breast cancer. Because it is so accurate and gives so much information, the CT scan is now more commonly used than the liver scan. It is very helpful in evaluating specific complaints in other parts of the body.

Every woman treated for breast cancer will look back as the years pass, and review her decisions in light of the eventual outcome. Throughout her life, every patient should continue to feel confident that she made the best possible treatment decisions for herself and her future.

The improved prognosis in many breast cancer cases stems mainly from earlier diagnosis and the use of adjuvant systemic therapies in almost every woman. Newer surgical treatments, although they don't improve prognosis, are far less disfiguring than older procedures.

† Local, Regional, and Adjuvant Treatment † Recommendations for Small (Under 2 cm) Invasive Ductal Breast Cancers

Of the various procedures available, only two—(1) modified radical mastectomy and (2) lumpectomy with removal of underarm lymph nodes and irradiation of the remaining breast tissue (breast conservation)—provide the best chance for complete treatment success. Either method is likely to effectively treat small cancers with minimal and equal chance of success. Even if I feel only one is appropriate, I discuss both options with my patients before giving my recommendation.

When Modified Radical Mastectomy Is the Treatment of Choice

Although modified radical mastectomy can be used to treat any type of breast cancer, I most often recommend it, instead of breast conservation, for women who:

- have large cancers

- have small breasts, so that their cancer is proportionately large in relation to breast size
- have a cancer just underneath the nipple/areola
- have additional intraductal cancer beyond the small invasive cancer
- have two cancers in the same breast, especially if they are not close together
- have cancer in both breasts (some women)
- are not interested in lumpectomy because they don't want to undergo four to six weeks of irradiation therapy
- state that they want "the therapy with the longest track record"

Mrs. Maryanne Morrison, age 57, came to see me for a second opinion after having had a biopsy that diagnosed ductal breast cancer. The biopsy had removed the cancer, but the pathology report stated that it had been two centimeters (¾ inch) in diameter. I noted the recent biopsy scar near the areola and felt no other lumps, no enlarged lymph nodes. Her mammogram, except for the cancer that had been removed, was normal.

Because of the location of the cancer and the small size of her breasts, I felt that mastectomy and reconstruction was the treatment of choice. To perform breast conservation would require removing the nipple, the areola, and almost all of the lower half of the breast.

Before giving her my recommendation, I described both procedures and then explained why I would not choose breast conservation. She told me that her surgeon had not even mentioned that option, merely stating that mastectomy was indicated. With all of the recent attention given to breast conservation, it is important for a woman to know why that option is not being offered to her.

WHEN LUMPECTOMY (BREAST CONSERVATION) IS THE TREATMENT OF CHOICE

I recommend breast conservation for many women with small breast cancers who:

- have a single cancer that is small in relation to breast size
- have cancers that aren't located under the nipple/areola
- express the desire to preserve as much of the breast as possible

Mrs. Lee Johns, age 40, had a very small lump, found only by mammography. Biopsy proved it to be invasive ductal cancer, the most common type of breast cancer. Because she met all the criteria for either breast conservation or modified radical mastectomy, I presented both options. I then explained that all of the data available to date show that the less extensive treatment, breast conservation, would be quite appropriate for her particular cancer.

She asked how doctors could recommend a treatment that had only been used for a relatively short time. I explained that the analysis of that data gives us every indication that the longer follow-up will be as good. That satisfied her and she opted for breast conservation.

OTHER TREATMENT OPTIONS

A very elderly or very ill patient who shouldn't undergo the strain of a modified radical mastectomy may elect to have a simple mastectomy or only a portion of breast conservation. A woman may also insist that her breast be left entirely intact, despite the indications for modified radical mastectomy or breast conservation; in this situation, irradiation therapy can sometimes be effective.

Above all, I make sure, before the woman makes her decision, that she understands all forms of treatment thoroughly—not only the procedures themselves but also their suitability for treating her particular cancer. There's no rush to decide, although I recommend letting no more than several weeks pass before scheduling the surgery, whichever it may be. If I think she may be a candidate for enrollment in a study of new breast cancer treatment, I discuss this possibility with her.

After all of the tissue is analyzed, I suggest that *every* patient seek consultation with an oncologist. She and the patient can discuss the pros and cons of adjuvant therapy and plan the best possible regimen.

† Local and Regional Treatment †
Recommendations for Intraductal
(Noninvasive) Breast Cancers

With very early cancers, mastectomy or breast conservation techniques usually provide equally good results. Since noninvasive cancers rarely, if ever, spread to the lymph nodes, there is little reason to remove them. Therefore the treatment options for this particular type of cancer are 1) simple mastectomy or 2) lumpectomy (without lymph node removal) followed by irradiation therapy.

If intraductal cancer is present in only one area, either treatment is excellent. But if it is more extensive and present in

several areas of the breast, simple mastectomy should be recommended. Oncologists rarely recommend adjuvant therapy
with these very early cancers.

† LOCAL AND REGIONAL TREATMENT †
RECOMMENDATIONS FOR LOBULAR
CANCER IN SITU

Because lobular cancer in situ is so poorly understood, both
diagnosing and treating it are difficult. This particular cancer
apparently does little harm if it is treated only by biopsy. But
a woman with this condition has a 5 to 10 percent chance of
already having an undiscovered invasive cancer in that breast.
And she has a 35 percent chance of later developing a different
invasive cancer in that breast or the opposite one.

Many surgeons recommend either a simple mastectomy or
a lumpectomy plus irradiation, as they would for an intraductal
cancer. Others do not feel any treatment is needed and recommend frequent breast examinations and mammography to
detect any developing cancer. Others advocate several random
biopsies of the breast to determine if any invasive cancer can
be found and, if not, careful and frequent screening. I believe
it is very important for any patient with lobular cancer in situ
to understand as much of this dilemma as possible before she
and I decide on her treatment.

The treatment of the other breast is even more controversial.
Because there is a high likelihood that invasive cancer will
arise in either breast at some future time, many physicians
and patients do not want to just wait for cancer to develop.

Some recommend bilateral preventative mastectomies. (See page 90.)

There is no universally accepted method of treatment for this condition. If the woman is willing to accept some risk, then it may be satisfactory to do frequent mammography and breast examinations (with or without the multiple biopsies), thus hopefully ensuring early detection of any invasive cancer that may develop. However, the surest way to avoid the potential danger is removal of the breasts—followed by immediate breast reconstruction.

Other factors must also be considered in making the difficult choice to undergo prophylactic mastectomy. Does the woman want to have children? If so, she may want to delay consideration of a prophylactic mastectomy because of her desire to nurse. Is she willing to accept the loss of nipple sensation (with a reconstructed breast) in exchange for peace of mind about her otherwise high risk of developing breast cancer?

Adjuvant therapy is generally not used in treating lobular cancer in situ.

Just recently, I was surprised when our pathologist phoned to inform me that the biopsy on Mrs. Barbara Allen, age 58, demonstrated fibrocystic changes *and* lobular cancer in situ. When she returned to my office later that day, I told her of the findings. We and her husband spent the next thirty minutes discussing her condition. It was obvious that we would need additional discussions, and I suggested they come back the following day.

By then Mrs. Allen was more composed and we essentially repeated our discussion of the previous day. Finally, she said that the

problem was just too complex for her to make a decision immediately. That was very appropriate, and we agreed to talk again in
a week when she returned to have her sutures removed.

In the end, she decided not to undergo any further treatment,
but to return frequently for examinations and mammography. But
she also asked whether she could change her mind if she found that
she could not live with this plan. I assured her that in that case I
would perform the bilateral preventative mastectomies and
reconstruction.

† LOCAL, REGIONAL, AND ADJUVANT TREATMENT †
RECOMMENDATIONS FOR SMALL (UNDER 2 CM)
INVASIVE LOBULAR BREAST CANCERS

Local treatment of small lobular cancers is typically the same
as for other small cancers—1) modified radical mastectomy
(with or without immediate reconstruction) or 2) breast conservation. However, the woman and her doctor must also
consider the 35 percent likelihood that invasive cancer might
occur in the opposite breast.

As for lobular cancer in situ, the three possible procedures
for the opposite breast are: very careful monitoring, multiple
biopsies of that breast, or prophylactic mastectomy. Even
when only one breast contains lobular cancer, the potential
for cancer in the opposite breast can never be ignored.

† LOCAL, REGIONAL, AND ADJUVANT TREATMENT †
RECOMMENDATIONS FOR LARGE (GREATER
THAN 2 CM) BREAST CANCERS

Local treatment of large breast cancers is based on the same
principles as those for treatment of small breast cancers. In

addition, almost *all* women with large breast cancers require adjuvant therapy.

Although some surgeons are recommending breast conservation for women with breast cancers up to four centimenters (one and one-half inches), especially when the breasts are large, most surgeons do not. All surgeons should consider each particular woman individually, but any cancer larger than four centimeters should almost always be treated by modified radical mastectomy, with or without reconstruction. If lobular cancer is diagnosed, then treatment of the other breast must be considered, as is discussed above.

† Local, Regional, and Systemic Treatment †
for Metastatic Breast Cancer

Complete cancer eradication is possible in few women with such advanced breast cancer. For most, treatment is directed at controlling the cancer and prolonging life as long as possible with as little disruption of daily life as possible. With the effective treatments available today, many women with metastatic breast cancer are going about their daily lives much as they did before.

Treatment to slow or stop the spread of cancer is even more urgent than the local/regional treatment of the breast itself. Increasingly women are deciding, with an oncologist's guidance, to begin a program of chemotherapy (sometimes in combination with hormonal and/or irradiation therapy) even before breast surgery is performed. The local/regional treatment is almost always a modified radical or simple mastectomy.

†

Mrs. Christine Frances, age 56, learned she had breast cancer only after investigation of a painful hip revealed it was the site of a metastatic lesion stemming from a cancer in her left breast. Her lymph nodes were also enlarged, and further testing showed other areas of cancer spread. She needed combination therapy: systemic chemotherapy to minimize further cancer spread, irradiation of the hip lesion, and treatment of the breast. Because we already knew she had metastatic disease, lymph node removal for staging was unnecessary. But removing them would decrease the amount of cancer left in the body. She agreed to undergo a modified radical mastectomy, which would quickly deal with the lesion in the breast, and then proceed with the rest of her therapy.

Some oncologists would begin adjuvant therapy and irradiation of the hip even before the mastectomy. Both methods have their advantages and each patient must be considered individually.

Treatment of a single known metastatic area may include irradiation therapy to eradicate the lesion at the new body site or at least slow its growth. Although chemotherapy and hormonal therapy can have a similar beneficial effect on individual cancer lesions elsewhere in the body, they usually respond best to direct irradiation therapy.

Systemic therapy, particularly chemotherapy, for metastatic cancer should begin as soon as possible. Combinations of chemotherapeutic drugs have been shown to induce therapeutic responses and even remissions in up to 80 percent of cases. However, because chemotherapy drugs and treatment regimens are constantly under review, a woman having chemotherapy should be continuously monitored by her oncologist to be sure she's receiving the most up-to-date and potentially effective treatment.

A *remission*, when all of the known cancer appears to be eradicated, may last for weeks, months, or years. If the cancer eventually begins to grow again, the treatment can often be changed, leading to another period of remission. A woman may experience a number of such cycles.

† RECOMMENDATIONS IF BOTH BREASTS † ARE FOUND TO CONTAIN CANCER

When cancer is present in both breasts, partial mastectomy (breast conservation) is less commonly recommended because of the extensive irradiation that would be needed to treat both breasts. Yet today some radiotherapists are beginning to treat such patients. Fortunately, it is unusual to discover breast cancer in both breasts at the same time. Most often, the surgeon recommends modified radical mastectomy on each side, with or without immediate breast reconstruction.

† LOCAL, REGIONAL, AND ADJUVANT TREATMENT † FOR INFLAMMATORY CANCER

These particular cancers carry the worst prognosis of any breast cancer and must be aggressively treated by combination therapy. The best results appear to occur when chemotherapy is used first, followed by irradiation therapy and surgery. There is extensive research being conducted on the treatment of inflammatory cancer, and the recommendations depend upon the individual circumstances.

† Recommendations for Treatment of a † Recurrence of the Cancer in the Remaining Breast Tissue or in the Mastectomy Site

The recurrence of a cancer in the local area of the breast poses a difficult problem. Not only must the woman deal with the need for additional treatment some time after her initial surgery, but she may also have a period of depression, knowing that her initial treatment was not totally successful and that she has cancer again.

If cancer is found in the breast after breast conservation, it can frequently be successfully treated by performing a mastectomy. If the cancer recurs after a mastectomy, but in the area of the mastectomy, then the usual treatment consists of surgically removing the cancer and/or treating that area with irradiation. If that is the only recurrence, treatment will hopefully be successful.

With any local recurrence, the use of chemotherapy or hormonal therapy should be strongly considered.

† Recommendations for Treatment of Recurrent † Disease Not in the Breast Area

The likelihood of complete eradication of a breast cancer that recurs is, unfortunately, low. But we are continually coming up with new and more effective treatments to slow its growth and to prolong life—and to enable women whose cancer has recurred to live full and satisfying lives. The woman, her doctor, and her oncologist work closely together to decide on the treatment plan. The oncologist usually becomes her primary physician at this point.

Irradiation therapy is very effective for advanced cancer that has spread to distant sites, such as bone. But it can only be used for one or at most a few body areas at a time. It can't be used to treat cancer that has spread throughout the body or to certain body areas. Should that occur, hormonal therapy and/or chemotherapy become the principal treatment. Each patient requires continual monitoring because improvements in these treatment regimens occur frequently.

† MANAGING POST-TREATMENT DISCOMFORT †
AND COMPLICATIONS

Any kind of surgery leaves some discomfort in its wake. In addition, breast cancer surgery can cause certain specific problems:

Bleeding. Bleeding from any operation, if it occurs, will almost always happen in the first twenty-four hours after surgery. Sometimes it can be stopped by putting pressure over the surgical area with a dressing, but other times it may require a second operation. It is rarely serious.

Infection. Even the best efforts to prevent infection of a surgical incision can fail; infection may set in a few days or so after the operation, necessitating more visits to the surgeon for antibiotics and sometimes additional minor surgery.

Arm swelling. When the lymph nodes are removed from the underarm area, 5 to 10 percent of women experience arm swelling. It is not dangerous, but it can be annoying and even painful.

Treatment consists first of simply "favoring" the arm during the worst of the swelling and elevating it at night. Often this simple regimen is effective, but if it isn't, the doctor may suggest wrapping the arm with an elastic bandage at night (and then during waking hours if necessary). It is unusual for the swelling to worsen despite such treatment, but if it does, the doctor may prescribe the use of a special support sleeve or a pressure pump on the arm for several hours each day while the woman is resting. The sleeve or pump helps push fluid out of the arm.

Arm swelling can occur soon after the surgery or months, even years, afterward. Fortunately, it doesn't usually signify cancer recurrence.

Numbness of the armpit, mastectomy area, and arm. Some degree of numbness always occurs in the armpit and in the skin remaining in the mastectomy area; it usually lessens after some months, but some is permanent. Numbness of the upper inner arm also may occur, but does so less often today because the surgeon can usually preserve the nerves going to the skin of that arm.

† LIFELONG FOLLOW-UP †

When a woman's initial treatment ends, a lifelong period of *follow-up* begins. One doctor on her treatment team should continue to see her for regular breast screening. As the surgeon, I do this for all the women I treat for breast cancer. I make sure a woman leaves my office after a follow-up examination with a card noting the date and time of her next appointment, or a reminder card if it's some months in the future. If she doesn't return when scheduled, we try to reach her to encourage continued follow-up evaluations with me or another physician of her choosing.

But her follow-up visits need not be limited to routine checkups. Anytime she has a concern, her physician must be available to answer her questions and see her if necessary.

When she returns for a checkup, I first question her regarding *any* complaints she may have, not only those related to the breast area. I need to determine if I should be suspicious of any area where a metastasis might be developing (usually in bone, lung, or liver). If a cancer is found in the opposite breast, it is almost always new, not spread from the first one.

I then ask her specifically about any discomfort in her back, arms, or legs; unexplained weight loss; coughing, hoarseness, or gastrointestinal disturbances; or lumps she may have noticed. And I always ask, "Is anything else bothering you?"

The site of the original cancer is first examined and then the other breast. If any suspicious area is noted, it must be fully investigated, and possibly biopsied.

Another essential ingredient of effective follow-up examinations is a yearly chest X-ray and a mammogram of the opposite breast, if a mastectomy was done; or of both breasts if a breast conservation procedure was performed.

† PREGNANCY AND BREAST CANCER †

Breast cancer usually but not always occurs after the reproductive years, and so it is not generally associated with pregnancy. But when it does occur in pregnant women, it requires special considerations.

Breast Cancer Discovered During Pregnancy

Fortunately, few pregnant women are diagnosed as having breast cancer. And there are few statistics that give us information on the number of women affected. A study reported from the Kaiser Permanente Medical Center in 1985 had 19 pregnant women among 1,400 who developed breast cancer— slightly over 1 percent. But of the 176 women of childbearing age, the same 19 women represented 11 percent. The study found their prognosis to be the same as for the similar group of nonpregnant women. Most surgeons do not routinely recommend terminating the pregnancy, unless extensive chemotherapy is warranted. But the question has never really been answered and each pregnant woman must be considered on an individual basis.[1]

Recently Mrs. Betty Witkin, age 26, came to see me with a newly discovered three-centimeter lump in her right breast. She immediately informed me that she was sixteen weeks pregnant and had two other children. Biopsy demonstrated ductal cancer and she had lymph nodes that were suspicious for cancer. She underwent a modified radical mastectomy with reconstruction. Five of her lymph nodes contained cancer, so she also needed adjuvant chemotherapy.

Most oncologists would be very hesitant to treat a woman in the second trimester of her pregnancy with the very toxic chemotherapy drugs, which are not approved by the FDA for use in pregnancy. I believe Mrs. Witkin had two options: either to continue the pregnancy and delay adjuvant therapy, or to terminate the pregnancy and begin the therapy immediately. She decided to have an abortion, so that the chemotherapy could be begun immediately.

Subsequent Pregnancy After Breast Cancer

In the past, physicians assumed that a pregnancy after cancer treatment might worsen a woman's prognosis, and they always strongly recommended that it be avoided. That recommendation was not based on sound scientific data, but rather on the knowledge that some breast cancers are stimulated by hormones such as estrogen and that the estrogen level is significantly increased during pregnancy. However, we now know that most women in their childbearing years do not have estrogen receptors in their breast cancer.

To date no studies have determined whether it is safe to become pregnant after having had breast cancer. In my practice, several women have successfully completed one or more pregnancies without any unusual occurrences.

In the mid-1970s, Ms. Dorothy Daniels, age 35, came in for a routine checkup, three years after being treated for a small breast cancer. She had had a modified radical mastectomy and more recently a delayed reconstruction. She informed me that she had married and wanted to have a child. I told her what I knew about the risks involved and said that I wanted to research the recent medical literature to see if there was anything new on that subject.

I reported back to her that there was *no* data that demonstrated any increased risk in her becoming pregnant and carrying her child to term. She decided to have a child and became pregnant within a year. Now, some ten years later, she and her daughter are doing very well. When she brings Betsy with her to my office, I am always reminded how careful physicians must be in giving advice, especially if it is not based on sound scientific data. Had I just recited the usual concerns about cancer and pregnancy to her, Betsy might not be here today.

A woman who wants to have a child after having been successfully treated for breast cancer should consider pregnancy only after all adjuvant therapy is completed and only if she has no known disease. She must understand that there is no absolute data which show that pregnancy is not dangerous. It is a decision she will have to make.

10

"What Are My Chances?"

Not every woman treated for breast cancer asks the question "What are my chances?" But I believe it's always foremost in a woman's thoughts. And her doctor's responsibility is to answer it as quickly, clearly, and accurately as possible. He can't answer it fully when the diagnosis is first made, but as the woman moves through diagnostic and treatment procedures, a detailed picture of her condition and chances for successful treatment emerges.

A woman's chances of surviving breast cancer can be deduced from the results of studies of thousands of women like her who have had breast cancer like hers. This statistic represents the percentage of women who have been treated successfully—that is, who have had no further problems with the disease over certain periods of time.

After surgery, analysis of the removed tissue gives a doctor the information she needs to estimate her patient's chances that the breast cancer will never recur. As a general and firm rule, the more a woman knows and understands about her disease, the better she'll cope with it.

Fortunately, most women have good to excellent chances for successful treatment if their cancer is discovered early. Although about 10 out of every 100 women will develop breast cancer, 9 of those 10 can be successfully treated *if the disease is detected early*, so 99 out of every 100 women need not die of breast cancer.

Treatment for breast cancer always involves surgery, and I am sometimes asked if that surgery will cause the cancer to spread. *It does not.* This erroneous belief apparently stems from the fact that in years past most breast cancers went undiscovered until they were very large. And we had fewer options for treating large cancers. So the mortality rate from the disease was high, not because of the surgery, but because the disease was already advanced by the time surgery took place.

Whether the outlook is excellent, good, fair, or poor, the percentage of successfully treated women in any group of women with breast cancer is only a guideline, because each woman responds differently to the disease and to treatment. Some women with a poor prognosis do remarkably well.

If I'm treating a woman for breast cancer and if her outlook for successful treatment appears poor, I make certain she and her family understand that they should never give up hope. After all, she may well fall into the statistical group of women like her, with breast cancer like hers, who never have problems with the disease again. And new drugs and procedures are being developed that improve the outlook for women with all types—and stages—of breast cancer.

With many types of cancer, a person may be considered "cured" after a certain period (five years is often used) of disease-free survival. Breast cancer, unfortunately, can never be spoken of as "cured." The disease may reappear at any time. True, this risk lessens with each year that passes without recurrence (after fifteen disease-free years, recurrence is extremely rare). But a woman who has had breast cancer must maintain personal vigilance and careful medical follow-up for the rest of her life.

† Is the Cancer Noninvasive † or Invasive?

Generally noninvasive cancers have the best outlook, but even small invasive cancers can have a favorable prognosis.

Mrs. Maureen Marsh, age 32, came to see me for the first time following referral by her gynecologist. She'd called him after noticing, while dressing, that she had a small lump just above the nipple of her right breast. When I examined the breast, I felt a very tiny lump (about three millimeters in diameter, less than one-quarter of an inch) just above the areola. My examination suggested it was probably a small, benign fibroadenoma, but I could not be sure, so I recommended a breast biopsy. The lump turned out to be intraductal cancer; almost certainly, no lymph nodes were involved. So Mrs. Marsh's chances for successful treatment were excellent. Over 95 percent of women with her breast cancer characteristics never have problems with the disease again.

After listening to my recommendations, she decided on a simple mastectomy with immediate breast reconstruction. There was no need for removal of lymph nodes, subsequent irradiation, or other adjuvant therapy. In the three years since her surgery, Mrs. Marsh has had no recurrence of her cancer.

Mrs. Eileen Jepson, age 60, first came to my office seven years ago after discovering a lump in her left breast. It was prominent (two centimeters in diameter, just under one inch), and a biopsy confirmed the diagnosis of invasive breast cancer. Today, I frequently recommend lumpectomy with removal of the lymph nodes and irradiation therapy for cancers like hers. But seven years ago, the treatment of choice was the one she decided on: modified radical mastectomy with immediate breast reconstruction. The lymph nodes did not contain cancer. From 70 to 80 percent of women with Mrs. Jepson's cancer characteristics never have problems with breast cancer again. Today, after seven years, she remains in this large, successfully treated group.

† SIZE OF THE CANCER †

In general, the smaller the cancer, the better the patient's chances for successful treatment. Fortunately, over the past few years, I've treated fewer women with large breast cancers. Most breast cancers are now discovered early through careful screening by women themselves and by their internists, family physicians, and gynecologists.

There is one exception to this generally positive trend. Sometimes I learn that a woman with a large breast lump first noticed it while it was still small but didn't seek medical attention until it became too large to ignore. This reaction is especially distressing because it prevents early treatment and because it compromises the chances that treatment will be successful.

Mrs. Ethel Dix, age 60, first came to see me about two years ago with a very large breast lump that proved to be cancer. In our subsequent discussions of her condition, I learned that she'd first noticed the lump over a year before, when it was much smaller, but had put off seeing a doctor about it "because I was afraid of what it would do to my marriage if it turned out to be breast cancer." After performing a needle biopsy, diagnosing breast cancer and discussing treatment, I explained to her that 60 to 70 percent of women with such large breast cancers have further problems with their disease.

As might be expected, Mrs. Dix reacted to this news with the same kind of fear that had apparently kept her from seeing a doctor when the lump was still small. But to my surprise, she also expressed relief at finally talking about it. And she was able to include her husband in our later discussions.

Mrs. Dix's delay in acknowledging to herself that she might have breast cancer is explainable, of course, in human terms. We all tend to block out fearful thoughts of disease and death in an attempt to postpone their arrival in our lives. However, Mrs. Dix's fear blocked her capacity for responding to even the physical signs of potentially life-threatening disease. As a result, although aggressive treatment has helped control her cancer for two years, she still has evidence of cancer in her body and her chance for a successful outcome of treatment is not good.

† INVOLVEMENT OF LYMPH NODES †

The best outlook occurs when no or at best just a few lymph nodes contain cancer.

I first met Ms. Janet Carson, age 45, sixteen years ago when she came to my office for examination of a lump about three centimeters (over one inch) in diameter in the mid-upper portion of her right breast. My examination also detected an extremely enlarged lymph node under the arm on the same side.

Her diagnosis and treatment followed the one-step pattern prevalent in those years. While she was under general anesthesia, the lump was removed and biopsied, and she was operated on immediately because the biopsy results were positive for cancer. I performed a modified radical mastectomy and also removed many large lymph nodes that I suspected were cancerous. (Usually a surgeon who removes possibly cancerous lymph nodes can't tell or even guess if they actually are, but her nodes were very suspicious.) The pathology report showed that of thirty-two nodes removed, twenty were cancerous.

After her surgery, Ms. Carson had chemotherapy and adjuvant irradiation therapy in the breast and armpit, as recommended by a consulting oncologist. Tests showed no apparent evidence of cancer elsewhere in her body. That was good news, but I still had to tell Ms. Carson that among women with breast cancer like hers, about 80 percent could expect the disease to recur at some time in the future. Of course, I also reminded her that she could well be in the second, smaller group—the long-term survivors.

And I'm glad I did. Sixteen years later, she *is* in that smaller group, and her odds against recurrence improve with the passing years. Every time I see her, I'm reminded of the uniqueness of each of my patients and of their potential to survive even when the odds are stacked against them.

† Has the Cancer Spread to † Distant Sites?

Today, we can control metastatic cancer growth better than ever before. As a result, the outlook for women with this stage of the disease can include months and years of disease-free remissions and productive living.

Sometimes—although much less often today than formerly—breast cancer has already spread to distant tissues by the time it's first discovered. Ms. Angela Marion, age 48, was referred to me by her gynecologist after he found a lump in her breast. It was fairly large (about four centimeters, or one and one-half inches, in diameter), and biopsy indicated it was cancer.

Before having the modified radical mastectomy with immediate reconstruction she'd decided on, Ms. Marion saw an oncologist for a second opinion. At his recommendation, she had a bone scan and a liver scan for detection of possible metastases. The bone scan showed that the cancer had spread to her lower spinal column.

After Ms. Marion's initial surgical treatment (which also revealed that some of her lymph nodes were cancerous), she started chemotherapy and received irradiation therapy in the affected area of her back.

That was a lot of therapy, but it apparently did a lot of good. For, eighteen months later, the cancerous area in her back hasn't flared up again, and although a new area in a rib has also been treated with irradiation therapy, Ms. Marion is getting along well and continuing to live and work much as she did before her cancer was discovered.

Angela Marion still has cancer, of course, and that won't change. But it's under control so far, and the fact that we can control it today gives us hope for controlling it tomorrow. Although her chances for living a full span of years are low, the constant flow of new drugs and technologies for treating cancer gives us hope.

† THE OUTLOOK FOR INFLAMMATORY CANCER †

Treatment for this uncommon but very aggressive cancer must include every possible form of therapy to improve a woman's rather poor chance of survival. Fortunately, some women beat those odds by a considerable margin.

About eight years ago, Mrs. Ellen Arnold, age 40, the sister of a close friend, was referred to me for examination of redness and irritation in her left breast. She hadn't yet had a mammogram. My examination revealed thickening of the skin of the left breast along with redness and enlarged pores. I was concerned that this was inflammatory breast cancer. An immediate mammogram showed no lump or other abnormality except skin thickening on the left breast, but a subsequent breast biopsy indicated she did have inflammatory cancer.

I explained that a woman with this type of breast cancer can only rarely expect treatment to be completely successful and that I wanted to obtain an immediate consultation with an oncologist.

As a result, over the next four months she received extensive chemotherapy and irradiation treatments. When these were completed, I biopsied the left breast again. The cancer, although now less extensive, was still present. Other studies had shown no evidence that it had spread (although I suspected it had), so she was determined to be a good candidate for a modified radical mastectomy. Afterward, she received more chemotherapy as well as hormonal therapy, and the right breast and other suspectible areas of her body were carefully checked at regular and close intervals.

For four years, Mrs. Arnold's cancer did not recur—a very good result. Then, during a routine checkup, she told me that several weeks earlier she had noted a little red spot on her other breast. I immediately biopsied the spot: it was inflammatory cancer.

After consultation with the oncologist, I performed a modified radical mastectomy to remove Ellen Arnold's right breast. Afterward, she received additional chemotherapy and hormonal therapy and entered on a period of two more symptom-free years. Finally, six years after the onset of her cancer, it spread to other areas of her body; after an additional eighteen months of extensive treatment, she died.

Although the outcome of her disease was eventually tragic, her story demonstrates the degree of life extension possible even when the outlook is poor. When her disease was first discovered, Ellen Arnold's daughters were ten and twelve years old; they were both in college when she died.

† Living with Breast Cancer †

At first, a diagnosis of breast cancer is a shock and a source of deep anxiety to the woman and her family and friends. After her initial treatment, however, her anxiety usually is replaced to some extent by the reassurance that something has been done, that she's doing well, and that the cancer's long-term threat has been minimized.

TABLE 10-1

Factors Affecting the Successful
Percentage of Women Who Can Expect

Type of Cancer	Size	How Discovered
NONINVASIVE	VERY TINY ⅛ inch or 3 to 4 mm	1. By mammography 2. Nipple discharge 3. Rarely felt
I N V A S I V E C A N C E R	MINIMAL smaller than ½ inch or 13 mm	1. By mammography 2. Sometimes felt
	SMALL ½ to 1 inch or 13 to 25 mm	1. Usually felt 2. Almost always seen on mammography
	LARGE 1 to 2 inches or 25 to 50 mm	1. Lump is felt 2. Seen on mammography
	VERY LARGE over 2 inches or 50 mm	1. Lump is felt 2. Seen on mammography
INFLAMMATORY CANCER	NO DEFINITE SIZE	1. Redness, swelling 2. Pain 3. Usually no lump 4. Skin swelling seen on mammography

But the anxiety doesn't ever go away completely, even if her likelihood of successful treatment is excellent. That's to be expected, and it's probably beneficial. It keeps her on the alert for signs of possible cancer recurrence, and usually keeps her returning to her doctor for routine follow-up visits.

In general, the women I've treated for breast cancer deal with their disease better and better as time goes on, although most feel a little nervous just before coming in for routine

Treatment of Breast Cancer
Never to Have Their Breast Cancer Recur

If No Lymph Node Involvement	*If Lymph Nodes Are Involved*
95% to 100% (most do not have lymph node involvement)	Similar to invasive cancer (rarely are lymph nodes involved)
80% to 95% (about ⅔ have no lymph nodes involved)	60% to 70% (about ⅓ have lymph nodes involved)
70% to 80% (about ½ have no lymph nodes involved)	60% if 1 to 3 involved nodes 40% if 4 or more involved nodes (about ½ have involved nodes)
50% to 70% (few do not have lymph nodes involved)	40% if 1 to 3 involved nodes 30% if 4 to 10 involved nodes 20% if more than 10 involved
Only a rare woman will not have involved lymph nodes	30% if 1 to 3 involved nodes 20% if 4 to 10 involved nodes 15% if more than 10 involved
Only a rare woman will not have involved lymph nodes	Less than 10% (most will have involved nodes)

checkups. For a few, however, anxiety about the threat of cancer recurrence remains at an uncomfortably high level for years after successful treatment.

During her first visit to my office, three years ago, Mrs. Joanne Sutter, age 46, was extremely anxious and upset. A biopsy performed elsewhere had confirmed that she had breast cancer. Despite her tears and my regret that nothing I said seemed to help, we got through that first conversation and those that followed, and she elected to undergo a lumpectomy with lymph node removal and follow-up irradiation therapy. I removed the breast cancer and was relieved to find that it was very small and noninvasive and did not involve her lymph nodes. Over 95 percent of women in her circumstances never have problems with breast cancer again.

She recovered quickly from the surgery, and, as expected, her cancer has not recurred. Nevertheless, until very recently she was just as anxious and upset every time I saw her as she was the first time. She'd calm down a little after a routine examination showed no evidence of cancer recurrence, but I was concerned that her anxiety might be affecting her ability to cope with the stress and strain of daily life.

This is a delicate situation for the doctor involved. How much should she inquire into the woman's emotional state? What recommendations can she make for her patient to get emotional support for a more positive outlook? Some women are offended or made more anxious by the suggestion that psychotherapy might help calm their fears and improve their spirits.

Over the years, I've found that most of my patients welcome information about support groups. These are groups of women with breast cancer who meet informally for mutual support and understanding. Although a professional therapist is usually involved in guiding such a group's discussions, the support mainly grows out of the therapeutic relationships that develop among the women.

I tried several times to interest Mrs. Sutter in joining such a group, with no success. But during her most recent checkup, she told me that a close friend had been diagnosed as having breast cancer and was "terribly upset" about it. She was so concerned about her friend, she explained, that she'd decided to join a support group with her. I was very glad to hear that. It meant that Mrs. Sutter was ready to put aside her own anxiety to help her friend. Almost certainly, that generous act would improve the outlook for both of them.

† A Final Word †

Of course, the best protection against anxiety and fear about breast cancer is our ever-improving ability to diagnose the disease (including recurrence) early enough for treatment to have the best chance for success. That's why regular checkups with the doctor (including mammography) and monthly breast self-examination are so important for all women, especially those who have had breast cancer.

But regular checkups provide other benefits as well. Facing the future with confidence and strength is a critical element in keeping breast cancer at bay, and the doctor is an important source of that confidence and strength for every woman with breast cancer. She needs (and should expect) her doctor's reassurance that she'll continue to see her for checkups throughout the coming years and be available for consultation without long waits for appointments.

11

A New Beginning:
Breast Reconstruction Surgery

Since 1976, I have recommended breast reconstruction for over 90 percent of my patients who have modified radical or simple mastectomies. Surgeons first began creating natural-looking breast mounds to replace breasts in 1971, and many thousands of women have opted to have this surgery as an immediate follow-up to all types of mastectomy or as a separate operation months or years later. There is no time limit.

Breast reconstruction isn't merely a cosmetic refinement, any more than an artificial limb can be considered cosmetic. An artificial limb makes the person whole again; so does a reconstructed breast. No one needs or deserves to be less than whole when a safe and proven alternative is available.

True, none of the reconstruction procedures we have today can *exactly* reproduce the beauty or the function of a natural breast. But for a woman neither can having no breast compare with having one—with looking and feeling entirely herself.

Of course, planning the most effective treatment for cancer comes first. But if a woman and her doctor have selected mastectomy as her best option for local treatment, then they should strongly consider breast reconstruction as part of the overall treatment plan.

The main goal of breast reconstruction surgery is the creation of a breast mound that closely matches the remaining natural breast in size, contour, and feel. If both breasts are reconstructed, the surgeon makes them as much alike as possible and of a size appropriate for the woman's size and body type.

Breast reconstruction offers many advantages. It is more real-looking under clothes. It is more comfortable than wearing a prosthesis inside a bra cup, and a woman need not worry about the prosthesis slipping in her bra or even out of her bra. Perhaps most important, the breasts feel more natural: her body moves much as it did before the cancer surgery, and she carries herself the same way, with no sense of being off balance. Having a breast where there would otherwise be none helps prevent the loss of self-esteem and sexual identity that some women suffer after mastectomy.

The advantages of having a reconstructed breast are so great that there are now almost no arguments against it. A few women will decide they simply don't want the surgery. Most often, however, the question is what kind of reconstruction and when.

<h3 style="text-align:center">† SAFETY †</h3>

A 1985 study of 185 women, whose immediate breast reconstruction was performed at Bryn Mawr Hospital in Pennsylvania and at Georgetown University in Washington, D.C., demonstrated that their reconstruction had no adverse effect on breast cancer survival or treatment results.[1] After reconstruction, adjuvant treatment (if indicated) can proceed in the usual way. Even irradiation will have little effect on the silicone prosthesis—which, in turn, does not interfere with the irradiation. If the reconstruction is done later as a separate operation, it should be planned after the period of most intensive chemotherapy and/or irradiation treatment has been completed. Usually hormonal therapy does not affect this timing.

† TIMING OF BREAST RECONSTRUCTION †

The timing of breast reconstruction has no effect on treatment of the cancer in the vast majority of women. In the past, some doctors suggested a two-year wait between mastectomy and breast reconstruction in case the woman developed local cancer recurrence that the immediately reconstructed breast might "hide." But there is no evidence that a recurrence has ever been hidden. The silicone prosthesis is always placed behind the muscle, a place where few recurrences occur. Furthermore, the two-year period is arbitrary, since cancer can recur at any time.

Immediate reconstruction does have some important advantages, however. First, it requires only one hospitalization and one convalescence, saving time, money, and discomfort. Second, the woman never has to experience not having a breast; she awakens from the anesthetic with a reconstructed breast. Third, at the time of the mastectomy, the chest skin is much looser than it will be later, so the reconstructive procedure may be simpler to perform.

I've known some doctors who recommend that women "live without a breast" for a while after a mastectomy before having breast reconstruction. They feel that this would make them "appreciate" the reconstruction more! What nonsense—no one should have to live with a problem that can be corrected.

Like many other doctors, I advocate immediate breast reconstruction for women whose prognosis is poor. Why? Because self-esteem and quality of life are just as important for these women—maybe more important.

A survey carried out in Los Angeles, Washington, D.C., and Philadelphia and reported in 1985 showed that women having immediate breast reconstruction had less psychological distress than women who delayed their reconstruction.[2]

Delay in performing the reconstruction may be advised when a breast cancer is large and involves extensive amounts of skin and/or muscle. Likewise, if a woman is undergoing extensive adjuvant therapies, reconstruction should be delayed until her general health will support the additional surgery. Delay may also be advised when a woman is having a difficult time coping with having breast cancer and needs all her energy to focus on planning her primary treatment. Delayed breast reconstruction is somewhat more difficult (in my opinion) than immediate reconstruction, but it doesn't usually detract from the final cosmetic results.

† TECHNIQUES OF RECONSTRUCTION †

The surgeon uses the woman's own skin and muscle, and often a silicone implant, to construct a breast mound whose outward appearance is that of a natural breast. Some women don't bother to have the nipple and areola reconstructed; for those who do, it is done a few months after the creation of the breast mound, using tissue from the woman's own body.

The surgeon—who may be the surgeon performing the modified radical mastectomy or a specialist in reconstructive/plastic surgery—must keep the reconstructive surgery as simple as possible and make sure the new breast will not impede current or future cancer treatment or interfere with breast cancer screening.

At first reconstruction was not feasible if the mastectomy involved removal of large amounts of skin and/or muscle. Then in 1977 doctors began moving portions of skin and muscle from the back to enlarge the chest muscles and cover larger silicone implants, making breast reconstruction possible for almost any woman.

At about the same time, a procedure moving tissue from the lower abdomen to create a new breast *without* the use of a silicone prosthesis was developed. The skin/muscle-expander technique was developed more recently and is used most often today.

The method of reconstruction is chosen according to the characteristics of each individual patient. Regardless of the surgical procedure used, a reconstructed breast usually doesn't assume its final shape and position until several months after the surgery. Initially a woman may be somewhat disappointed, but if she has been properly prepared for the procedure, she'll know that the final result may be very different.

† Subfascial Reconstruction †

This comparatively simple and rapid operation can be done either immediately after a mastectomy or, less commonly, some time (even years) afterward. If it is done immediately, no additional incision or scar results, but even with later reconstruction, the incision can usually be made in the old mastectomy scar.

The surgeon constructs a pocket under the chest-wall muscles to hold the silicone implant, which he then covers with the skin and muscle remaining after the mastectomy. Over a period of months, the reconstructed breast mound becomes increasingly natural-looking. This type of reconstruction is usually used in relatively small-breasted women who have adequate skin and muscle to cover a silicone implant of the required size. For a few women, it produces an excellent-appearing breast; for most, one of the other methods will generally produce better results.

† Latissimus Muscle Transfer †

This procedure can be used for immediate or later breast reconstruction. It is especially useful for women whose remaining chest skin after mastectomy is insufficient to cover even an expander filled with very little fluid. It is also frequently used for later breast reconstruction in women who had full (Halsted) radical mastectomies to replace the pectoralis muscle that was removed.

The latissimus muscle is a large muscle on the upper back.

This operation moves a portion of that muscle, and sometimes skin from the back, to the chest. When done at the same time as the mastectomy (immediate reconstruction), an additional sixty to ninety minutes are required. When performed at a later time, several hours are needed. It is considered the best method available for transferring skin to the breast area, and the results can be excellent. Taking skin and muscle from the back causes no loss of function in that area. (See Diagram 11-1.)

† TRANSVERSE RECTUS ABDOMINAL FLAP TRANSFER †

In this procedure, the surgeon transfers skin, fatty tissue, and muscle from the lower abdomen to the mastectomy area. Usually this tissue is sufficient for the surgeon to create the new breast mound *without* a silicone implant. The cosmetic result is typically excellent. However, this procedure takes from three to five hours and is therefore most commonly used for delayed reconstruction surgery.

Because it requires an incision across the woman's lower abdomen and partial removal of skin and fatty tissue there, she receives the "bonus" of a tightening of the remaining abdominal skin and muscles. Thus, the transverse rectus transfer procedure is particularly appropriate for a woman who is slightly overweight and has some loose or flabby skin on her lower abdomen.

Of the available procedures, this is the one with the highest incidence of post-operative complications, including weakness

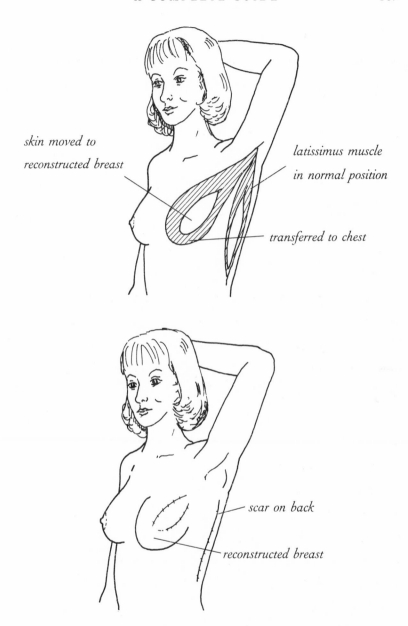

skin moved to reconstructed breast

latissimus muscle in normal position

transferred to chest

scar on back

reconstructed breast

DIAGRAM 11-1 Reconstruction Using Latissimus Muscle and Skin Transfer

or hernia of abdominal muscles and failure of some of the skin/muscle transfer to "take" in its new site. When the latter occurs, healing of the reconstructed breast may be delayed but usually requires no further surgery. (See Diagram 11-2.)

† SKIN AND MUSCLE EXPANDERS †

The most common method of breast reconstruction surgery involves the use of a temporary expandable implant to stretch the skin and muscle. The initial operation, to insert the temporary expandable implant under the woman's chest skin and muscle at the mastectomy site, can be done anytime after the breast is removed, but is particularly well suited to immediate reconstruction. Then, over a period of weeks or months, the implant is slowly expanded with periodic injections of salt water through a special valve on the expander—typically two to three ounces at a time, at two- to four-week intervals. This slowly stretches the skin and muscle until the mound is large enough to accommodate the insertion of a permanent implant of the desired size. (Usually the temporary implant is expanded until it's somewhat larger than the permanent implant; that way, the silicone prosthesis will move naturally under the skin in the slightly larger pocket.)

Skin and muscle expanders don't damage the woman's skin, because it is stretched slowly, just like the skin over a pregnant woman's enlarging uterus. Nor are the periodic injections uncomfortable, although the doctor can withdraw some fluid and expand more slowly if the woman complains of too much tightness. (See Diagram 11-3 and 11-3A.)

This technique offers another advantage when the expand-

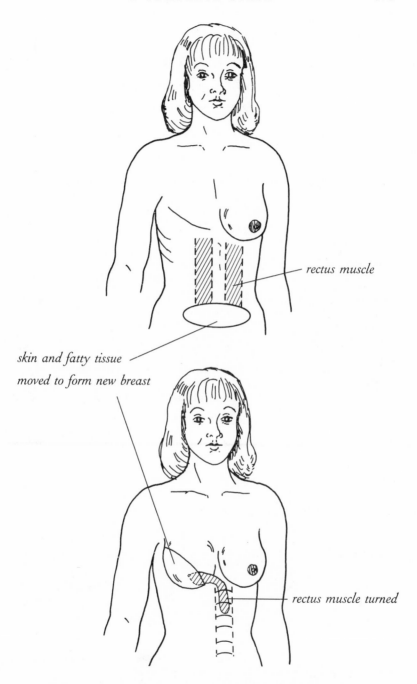

rectus muscle

skin and fatty tissue
moved to form new breast

rectus muscle turned

DIAGRAM 11-2   Transverse Rectus Abdominal Flap Transfer

able implant is removed and the permanent one inserted. The surgeon can then open or partially remove the tissue capsule (which always grows around an implant), allowing the implant to settle lower on the woman's chest with more natural-looking droopiness. In addition, the surgeon may make a small tuck in the skin below the reconstructed breast to form a more defined inframammary fold. This replacement of the expander is done under general anesthesia. It usually takes about thirty to forty-five minutes, and the woman can go home several hours later. During this second stage, an operation is sometimes performed on the opposite breast to provide greater symmetry. (See page 190.)

Some surgeons prefer to use a "permanent" expander, with a silicone outer layer, which is stretched to the desired size with salt water and then left in place. In this case, the second operation consists only of a small incision, using local anesthesia, to remove the implant's injection valve. Nothing is done to the capsule at that time; if it needs to be removed, an additional operation is scheduled.

† MICROVASCULAR TISSUE TRANSFER †

The secret to transferring tissue from one part of the body to another is maintaining the circulation to that tissue. The blood vessels have to remain connected or new connections must be made. The latissimus transfer and the transverse abdominal transfer *maintain the connections* already established. Microvascular tissue transfer *establishes new connections* by sewing the blood vessels attached to the skin and fatty tissue being

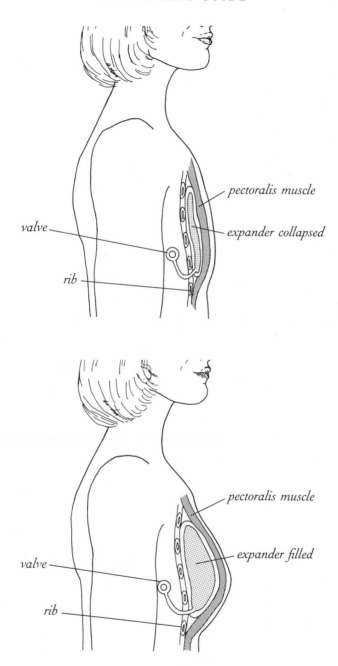

DIAGRAMS 11-3 and 11-3A   Skin/Muscle-Expander Technique

moved to the blood vessels already in place in the breast area.

This is a very delicate and long operation. It is not generally used for immediate reconstruction, although it can be. The tissue is frequently taken from the lower part of the buttocks or the lower abdomen, leaving a barely visible scar. It is then moved to the breast area and shaped to match the other breast, and the blood vessels are sewn together under an operating microscope. Still considered somewhat experimental, this very new procedure is now being performed in a number of medical centers in the United States.

† Nipple and Areola Reconstruction †

Many women don't bother to have this separate procedure performed, but some do. For a woman who does want nipple and areola reconstruction, the operation is done after the reconstructed breast has assumed its final shape and position—usually several months later.

Formerly, to reconstruct the areola, the surgeon used a graft of skin from the woman's groin crease—a slightly pigmented area that usually provides a good match for the areola on the remaining breast.

Most commonly now, a flap of skin is elevated from the breast mound and molded to create a nipple. The area exposed by the removal of the flap of skin is covered with a skin graft from any suitable area on the body. This elevated tissue and the skin graft are later tattooed to match the color of the opposite nipple and areola.

In the past the original nipple and areola from the cancerous breast were occasionally saved and put back on the breast. This technique was quickly discarded because of the danger of transplanting cancer cells into the reconstructed breast.

† What Happens to the Other Breast? †

Breast reconstruction attempts to create a new breast mound that looks as much like the remaining breast as possible. That can't always be done, however, particularly if the remaining breast is very large and droopy. In these circumstances, the reconstructive surgeon will probably recommend surgical lifting or reduction in size of the remaining breast to make it appear more like the reconstructed one. Surgery on the remaining breast takes place sometime after the breast reconstruction, possibly when an expander is changed for the permanent prosthesis.

Many women facing this decision simply don't want anything done to the remaining breast, so they decide they can live with less than ideal symmetry. For women who do opt for the additional surgery, these are the options:

· mastopexy (breast lifting) to correct droopiness
· reduction mammoplasty to make the remaining breast smaller
· augmentation mammoplasty to make the remaining breast larger (see page 186 for an explanation of why I don't recommend use of a silicone implant—required for augmentation mammoplasty—in the remaining breast of a breast cancer patient)

• prophylactic mastectomy and reconstruction of the remaining breast—occasionally a very reasonable choice for
a woman at high risk of developing cancer in the other
breast. Reconstructing both breasts allows achievement
of better symmetry.

† POSSIBLE COMPLICATIONS †

With any type of surgery, post-operative bleeding or infection may occur and require treatment. With breast reconstructive surgery, a portion of the skin and/or muscle covering
the silicone implant occasionally fails to survive after becoming infected or losing its blood supply. This is more likely to
occur in women who smoke, because smoking decreases blood
circulation even more. Usually only a small amount of skin
or tissue is lost, nothing happens to the prosthesis, and the
incision eventually heals. In about one woman out of fifty,
the complication is more serious and the implant may have
to be removed; it can usually be reinserted once the problem
is corrected.

I am sometimes asked if the prosthesis can break if the
woman has an accident. This almost never happens and if it
does, the silicone stays within the capsule surrounding the
implant.

Sometimes a woman isn't satisfied with the ultimate appearance of her reconstructed breast and just doesn't want to
"bother" with it. Removing the implant is a simple procedure
and the woman is no worse off than if she hadn't had the
reconstruction.

† Planning the Surgery †

My recommendation for immediate, or delayed, breast reconstruction takes place during my discussion of the patient's primary breast cancer treatment. This discussion frequently takes more than one visit to my office.

The surgeon performing a mastectomy may or may not also do breast reconstruction. If he doesn't, the treating surgeon will recommend a reconstructive surgeon to create the new breast. The patient must also meet him before the mastectomy to learn all the details and options that apply to her situation. She may even seek a second opinion from another reconstructive surgeon.

Mrs. Patricia Ellison was close to 40 when I performed a biopsy that indicated she had breast cancer. We met to plan her treatment and decided she was not a candidate for breast conservation. I recommended modified radical mastectomy followed by immediate breast reconstruction.

Like many women suddenly confronted with breast cancer, Mrs. Ellison knew little about breast reconstruction surgery. I explained the advantages along with the risks and possible complications, and then I showed her slides of women with reconstructed breasts of a size and type similar to her own. She agreed that there might be significant advantages for her in having her breast reconstructed. But she wanted to get more information and give the matter more thought before making a decision.

Three days later I marveled at how much she'd done and learned since our previous discussion. She'd consulted an oncologist for a second opinion, and spent hours at the local library reading the latest information available. Now she'd come to tell me that she agreed with my recommendation and would have her breast reconstructed.

This decision wasn't as straightforward as it sounds, because the oncologist had asked her why she wanted reconstruction, implying that she didn't "need" it. Of course, this was true from a medical standpoint, but his comment didn't take her present and future feelings about her body into account. Fortunately, she made her own decision with confidence.

I consider breast reconstruction (along with breast conservation) one of the most rewarding developments we've seen in the treatment of breast cancer. It enables the woman whose cancer is treated by mastectomy to have a normal-appearing figure that looks good and feels right for her body. She can wear any type of clothes without concern, from low-cut formal gowns to bikinis. And as a 68-year-old patient recently told me, "I swim every day and dress and undress with the other ladies. I really feel good about myself and am so pleased that I had reconstruction."

† WHAT A WOMAN NEEDS TO KNOW WHEN † CONSIDERING BREAST RECONSTRUCTION SURGERY

You should expect your doctor to cover each of the following points:

- The advantages, disadvantages (if any), and options for breast reconstruction.
- What's involved in immediate versus delayed reconstruction if you are currently deciding on primary treatment.

- The first reconstructive procedure involves creation of the breast mound. Creation of a nipple and areola, if desired, is done as a separate procedure at a later date.
- Some plastic surgery may be needed on the remaining breast to achieve symmetry with the reconstructed one.
- Various reconstructive procedures are available; why is one recommended over the others? (This should include a description of how the surgery will affect the woman's appearance both clothed and unclothed.)
- What the final breast will look like, using photographs of women whose breasts he has reconstructed to illustrate typical results of the surgery.
- If a second surgeon is needed to do the reconstruction, your doctor should refer you to a plastic reconstructive surgeon for consultation and planning before the mastectomy.
- If the doctor will be doing both the mastectomy and the reconstruction, he should offer you an opportunity to seek a second opinion from another reconstructive surgeon before making your decision.

Changing the Look of Your Breasts: Enlargement, Reduction, and Breast Lift Surgery

† BREAST ENLARGEMENT †
(AUGMENTATION)

Breast enlargement surgery is most often done for cosmetic reasons, to bring the woman's body proportions closer to what she considers normal for her and to improve her appearance. But cosmetic is not synonymous with frivolous. Over the past twenty-five years, this form of plastic surgery has become commonplace. Today, more than one million women have larger breasts thanks to this relatively simple and highly successful operation and most are very pleased with the results.

But are the breasts really larger? Yes and no. The breast mounds are two to four times larger, because the silicone implants placed beneath them (or beneath the pectoralis chest muscles underlying the breasts) add to the overall size. But the breast tissue itself is not enlarged: it is simply pushed outward by the implant. (Diagrams 12-1, 12-1A, 12-2, and 12-2A.)

The implant is a plastic sac, usually filled with silicone, a jellylike substance, or with salt water and silicone. The implant gives the enlarged breast a pleasingly symmetrical, natural-

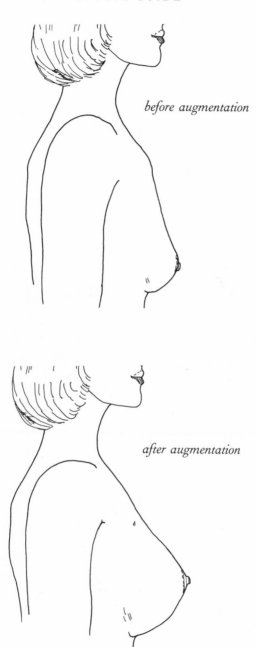

before augmentation

after augmentation

DIAGRAMS 12-1 and 12-1A   Breast Enlargement Surgery

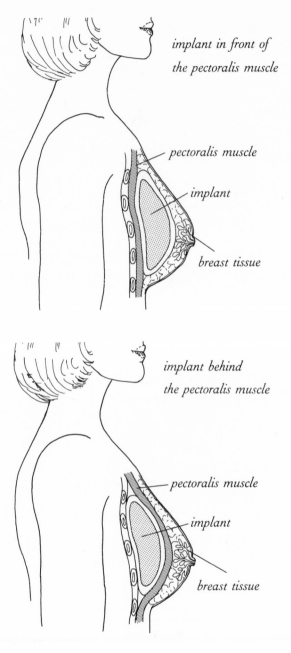

*implant in front of
the pectoralis muscle*

pectoralis muscle

implant

breast tissue

*implant behind
the pectoralis muscle*

pectoralis muscle

implant

breast tissue

DIAGRAMS 12-2 and 12-2A   Breast Enlargement Surgery

looking appearance and feel. The required incision may be in one of several different places on the breast and should be barely noticeable after it has healed.

FIRST STEP: CONSULTING WITH THE PLASTIC SURGEON

A woman thinking of having her breasts enlarged needs to understand (1) what her breasts will look like after the operation, (2) the surgical procedure to be used, (3) the types of side effects or complications that can occur and her chances of developing these problems, and (4) her specific reasons for having the operation. (For example, if she's anticipating a major change in her psychological outlook as a result of having larger breasts, she'll probably be disappointed—an outcome both she and the surgeon would want to avoid.)

A plastic surgeon may show a woman what to expect in a number of ways. She may use diagrams or photographs of women before and after the operation; some surgeons are using computer graphics. She will explain to her patient that it will be weeks or even months before the breasts and the implants "settle" into their final appearance.

Two different operations can be used to enlarge the breasts: placing the implant either behind or in front of the pectoralis muscle. Each method has its advantages. If the implant is placed behind the muscle, the operation is somewhat more difficult, but there is less likelihood of a thick capsule being formed and the enlarged breasts will appear more rounded. It is simpler to place the implant in front of the muscle, but the capsule may be more bothersome. Greater projection of the breast can be expected, however.

Each woman and her plastic surgeon must take the time to discuss the various options. If one operation was far superior to any other, we would all use it. But every woman is unique and what is correct for one might not be for another.

This surgery can't be expected to effect a "miraculous transformation" in the woman's self-image. She may, however, feel more attractive and comfortable about her appearance with larger breasts that have pleasing, symmetrical contours, look natural, and improve the fit of her clothes.

Surgery cannot enlarge a woman's breasts hugely. The plastic surgeon should explain the degree of enlargement the woman can reasonably expect. It can't significantly decrease the degree of natural sagging of the breasts that almost every woman eventually experiences, so sometimes enlargement surgery is combined with mastopexy. (See page 194.)

The surgeon should explain that the breast enlargement can be reversed and the woman's breasts restored to their former appearance, if that is ever desired. Although in theory this seems easy, it may require more extensive surgery. And once the implants are removed the breasts may not return to their original contours.

Considering the Complications

Understanding potential complications is particularly important because breast enlargement is cosmetic surgery—surgery that the patient does not absolutely need. A woman electing to have her breasts enlarged is also electing to take the risks associated with the surgery.

Bleeding. Excessive bleeding is unusual after this type of surgery, but it can happen and may necessitate a return to the operating room so it can be controlled.

Infection. Any surgery carries the risk of infection. Fortunately, it occurs in only about 1 percent of breast enlargement operations. When it does, the woman will need strong antibiotic therapy. Occasionally, the implant must be removed and replaced at a later date.

Capsule formation. Scar tissue, or a capsule, develops around every breast implant. Usually it is soft, so the woman won't even notice it. But occasionally, in one or both enlarged breasts, the capsule becomes tight and hard, making the breast feel unnaturally firm and distorting its contour. To treat this problem, the outside of the breast can be squeezed and manipulated by the surgeon to break up and soften the capsule (closed capsulotomy). In other cases, a simple surgical procedure may be needed to remove or open a part of the capsule. Some surgeons, at the time of surgery, use steroid drugs in or around the implant to minimize the likelihood of capsule formation, but that treatment is still experimental and not yet proven to be effective. We can't predict who will have problems with capsule formation, although research is ongoing. In addition, new implants are being developed to combat this problem.

Delayed detection of breast cancer. The most serious consequence of breast augmentation has been discovered only recently. It is not a complication of the surgery but a direct
result of having a silicone or salt water implant behind normal
breast tissue. The implants always cover some of the tissue,
so *mammography can't "see" into part of the breast.* (See Diagram
12-3.) The implant appears on every mammogram, regardless
of the angle it's taken from. No method of mammography yet
developed can entirely overcome this effect, although radiologists have developed techniques of mammography whereby
the breast is pulled or pinched in front of the implant so that
more of it can be seen on the X-ray picture.

Concealed from the mammographic "eye," early cancerous
changes may go undetected until the cancer has progressed
to a larger, more advanced, less curable stage. A study from
Van Nuys and Los Angeles, California, by a group of plastic
surgeons showed that *none* of twenty "augmented women"
who developed breast cancer between 1981 and 1986 had their
cancer found early by mammography alone. This contrasted
with the women without breast enlargement, a significant
number of whom had their breast cancer discovered very early
by mammography.[1] Breast enlargement surgery *doesn't cause*
breast cancer, but there is no doubt that it can delay its
diagnosis.

Although we have no good study similar to the one described above, it appears that the type of irregular and firm
capsule that forms around some implants may also delay the
finding of a lump by palpation.

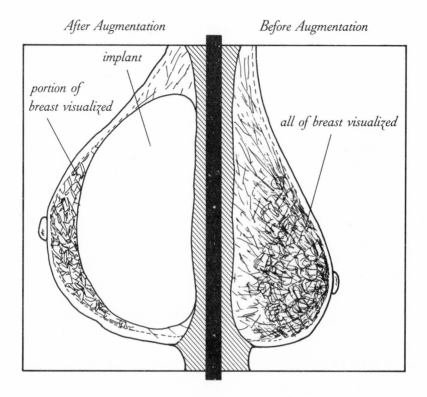

After Augmentation   *Before Augmentation*

implant

portion of
breast visualized

all of breast visualized

DIAGRAM 12-3   Mammogram with Silicone Prosthesis

Most women who have breast enlargement surgery are in their 20s or 30s. The first generation of women who have had their breasts enlarged are only now reaching their 40s and 50s, when both breast cancer and the practice of having regular mammograms are more common. As a result, these risks weren't discovered and publicized earlier.

Two of my colleagues from Washington University School of Medicine and Barnes Hospital in St. Louis, Drs. Judy Destouet and Leroy Young, have begun to search for a solution to this distressing problem. They are looking for other types of prostheses that might not interfere with mammography. At present their work is in the early stages, but they have discovered that prostheses filled with peanut oil do not seem to interfere with mammography. Their research has not yet entered the stage of testing on humans. Even if this is not the final answer, an acceptable implant will eventually be discovered.

If you have breast enlargement surgery, you have even more reason to have regular follow-up examinations with your physician and to maintain vigilant screening for any changes in your breasts.

Here are the main points to remember:

- See your doctor every six months for a thorough breast examination.
- If you're over 35, have a mammogram every year; the radiologist should take views from several angles in order to see more of the breast tissue. The radiologist will pull the breast tissue forward, away from the prosthesis, to include more of the breast tissue on the mammogram.
- If your doctor advises you to have a breast biopsy to rule out cancer, don't be afraid that this minor surgical procedure will "undo" your breast enlargement surgery. Most often the implant is left undisturbed, and it can be replaced immediately if any damage occurs.
- Examine your own breasts every month, especially if you have some degree of capsule formation around the im-

plant. Learn what the implant and capsule feel like. You will be in an excellent position to spot any changes.

A Nonproblem

The safety of having a silicone implant has recently been questioned. Experiments were reported in 1988 which showed that if rats had silicone injected beneath their skin, a type of rat cancer would develop. These cancers were not breast cancers. But researchers wondered whether silicone would also cause cancer in women's breasts. Many women with silicone implants asked me what they should do. I explained that cancer has never been found to be more prevalent in women with silicone implants. I would expect that if a connection existed, evidence would have shown up in the twenty-five years during which these implants have been used in over a million women.

Furthermore, the Food and Drug Administration issued a Drug Bulletin in 1989 reassuring us that the "study results are unlikely to be applicable to humans" and "if such an effect did exist, the risk would be very low."[2]

Cost of Breast Enlargement

The total cost of this operation will be over $2,000 and sometimes considerably more. Because it is cosmetic surgery, breast enlargement is not covered by any of the usual types of medical insurance, so the patient is responsible for paying the entire surgical fee and all the hospital and other costs involved, including the cost of the implants themselves.

† Breast Reduction †

Very large breasts are not as highly desirable in our society as some of the media would have us believe. The consequences of living with them are not all pleasant. Some women believe that large breasts are too conspicuous; they would like to feel less self-conscious about their appearance. Still others have a difficult time finding clothes that fit well, and some athletic women with large, bouncy breasts feel that smaller breasts would better suit their lifestyle.

There are also medical reasons for breast reduction. Large breasts are heavy; their weight pulls the woman's upper body forward and this can cause posture problems (a hunched-over, round-shouldered look) as well as neck and back pain. The pull of large breasts produces bra-strap grooves in a woman's shoulders. These can become unsightly and even painful. Skin irritation between and under large breasts can be a problem.

A woman who has had breast reconstruction following mastectomy may elect to have the remaining natural breast reduced to the same size as the reconstructed one. In some young women, one breast may become much larger than the other. These women may elect to have the larger breast reduced.

What's Involved in Breast Reduction Surgery?

Besides reducing the size of a woman's breast, reduction mammoplasty recontours them so they have a symmetrical and attractive appearance. Reduction mammoplasty can be accomplished by a number of different surgical techniques.

All the operations remove breast skin and breast tissue and usually move the nipples and areolae to a higher location. The amount of reduction necessary and the degree to which a woman's breasts droop determine the type of reduction mammoplasty used. (Diagrams 12-4 and 12-4A.)

Deciding to have breast reduction surgery involves the same basic steps as breast enlargement. The woman's conference with the plastic surgeon should include a realistic discussion of the benefits she can expect from having smaller breasts. She also needs to know the details of the surgical procedure, its possible side effects, and the expected appearance of the breasts after the operation.

No Effect on Early Detection of Breast Cancer

Although breast enlargement surgery has been shown to interfere with our ability to detect early breast cancer by mammography, breast reduction surgery appears to have no such effect. Scarring from breast reduction may make breasts more difficult to examine, but no proof exists that breast reduction delays the detection of any breast cancer.

Complications

Scarring. The surgery leaves scars at the incision sites on the breasts and around the areolae. These scars often widen over time and become more "feelable" and noticeable than the scars of breast enlargement surgery. The patient must understand that this occurs despite the plastic surgeon's best efforts to minimize the scarring through careful wound closure.

large pendulous breasts—before reduction

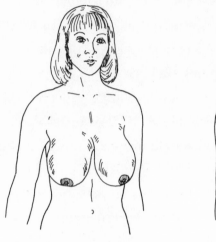
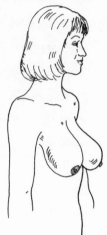

typical scarring from breast reduction

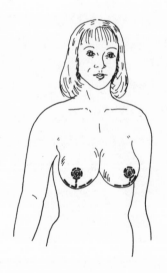
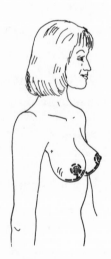

DIAGRAMS 12-4 and 12-4A   Breast Reduction Surgery

Everyone gets scars from surgery; the difference is that some people's bodies "heal better." Most women who have had this operation are pleased with the results and the scars are quite acceptable.

Decreased nipple sensation. This occurs with many techniques used for breast reduction. If nipple stimulation is very important sexually to a woman, she may decide against breast reduction surgery. Unfortunately, nipple stimulation may also become uncomfortable, although this is rare.

Loss of the ability to nurse. In many breast reduction operations, milk ducts leading from the breast glands to the nipple are cut and become nonfunctional, making nursing difficult or impossible. The functional loss can occur even if the ducts are not cut.

Surgical complications. As with breast enlargement, bleeding and infection can complicate breast reduction surgery. There is also a special complication: part of the flap of skin and tissue that is moved from its original site may die through loss of circulation. This condition is called *necrosis*. In its most serious and, fortunately, rare form, the nipple and areola do not survive. When necrosis occurs, surgical removal of the dead tissue is usually necessary. This causes more scarring, which may be helped by later plastic surgery.

WHAT IF THE RESULT ISN'T COMPLETELY SATISFACTORY?

Every surgeon who performs breast reduction surgery is careful to describe in detail all the things that can go wrong, including the fact that, even with his best efforts, he can't guarantee what the woman's new, smaller breasts will look like. Here are some of the problems that may occur during the months when the breasts are settling into position after the surgery:

- The woman may feel that her breasts are still too large, or she may be unhappy with the way they droop after surgery.
- The nipple and areola may be out of position on one or both of a woman's breasts.
- The breasts may not be as symmetrical in appearance as the woman wants them to be.
- There may be more scarring than the woman expected.

Sometimes these difficulties can be corrected or improved by additional surgery. If the woman is not pleased, she should speak frankly with her plastic surgeon and/or seek a second opinion.

COST OF REDUCTION MAMMOPLASTY

The cost of breast reduction surgery is similar to that of breast enlargement surgery, usually over $2,000 for the entire procedure. This operation, unlike breast enlargement surgery, is often covered by insurance. The plastic surgeon may have to send a letter to the insurance company to explain why this is not cosmetic but medically indicated surgery.

† MASTOPEXY (SURGERY TO LIFT THE BREASTS) †

Every woman's breasts undergo changes throughout her life. One such change is ptosis (sagging or droopiness), a natural consequence of growing older and having larger breasts. In addition, during pregnancy and nursing, the fluid and milk temporarily enlarge the breasts and stretch the skin covering them. When they return to their natural size, the skin tends to remain looser, for an overall sagging effect.

Of course, women vary in the degree of breast sagging; it is highly noticeable in some women, much less in others. But it happens to every woman, and there isn't much she can do to slow or stop it. Wearing a bra (especially during exercise) may help reduce the pull of the breasts on supporting tissues, but, in the long run, nature always wins out.

We do have a way to restore a more youthful look to sagging breasts, however: an operation called *mastopexy*. The surgery is similar to that for breast reduction, but the woman's breasts are not changed appreciably in size. Instead, the surgeon removes some breast skin to tighten the skin envelope around the breasts and lift them higher on the woman's chest. The nipples and areolae are also moved to a higher position.

The term *mastopexy* actually encompasses a number of surgical procedures for lifting the breasts; as with the other types of breast surgery I've discussed, a woman's surgeon will recommend and describe the specific procedure he believes is best for her.

WHAT THE WOMAN CONSIDERING MASTOPEXY NEEDS TO KNOW

The woman considering mastopexy, like the woman considering breast enlargement or reduction, should have a lengthy and detailed discussion with the plastic surgeon before making her decision. Because mastopexy is technically similar to breast reduction surgery, the possible complications are basically the same, including scarring (see page 191).

There is one major difference with mastopexy, however: the results are often not permanent. The woman needs to understand that although this operation can temporarily alter the natural process of skin aging, her breasts may eventually sag again.

MASTOPEXY OF THE OPPOSITE BREAST AFTER MASTECTOMY

The vast majority of women who undergo mastopexy do so for cosmetic reasons. They want breasts with more firmness and uplift. But there is a group of women for whom mastopexy is *not* cosmetic surgery: women who have had one breast removed and reconstructed because of breast cancer. Usually, the reconstructed breast has more uplift than the remaining, natural breast, and the only way to create symmetry is to correct the sag of the natural breast by mastopexy.

Medical insurance companies sometimes need to have this explained before they will cover the expense of the mastopexy, for generally it is not covered. Here is a sample of the kind of letter I write for my patients:

To Whom It May Concern:

Ms. —— is a 52-year-old woman who two years ago was diagnosed as having cancer of the right breast. She had a modified radical mastectomy and reconstruction using an expander, which was replaced with a permanent prosthesis eighteen months ago.

The reconstructed breast is the proper size, but the next step in completing the reconstruction will be to perform a mastopexy on the left breast to make the two breasts as symmetrical as possible. Ms. ——— is now ready and able to undergo that procedure; she asked me to write this letter so that you could review the situation and determine that this is, indeed, the next step in the reconstruction and should be a covered expense.

IF YOU'RE CONSIDERING SURGERY TO CHANGE THE LOOK OF YOUR BREASTS

As I explain to all my patients, the decision to have any operation—even for serious medical conditions—must be made carefully and with full consideration of all the possible problems as well as the benefits. With surgery such as breast enlargement, breast reduction, or mastopexy, the decision to expose oneself to surgical risks assumes even greater importance. Before deciding to have surgery to change the look of your breasts, get all the information you can, the negative as well as the positive. You will then be in a position to make an informed decision.

Notes

2. Your Guide to Breast Screening

1. Sam Shapiro, M.D. "Determining the Efficacy of Breast Cancer Screening." *Cancer* 1989, 63:1873–1880.
2. Charles M. Huguley, M.D., Robert Brown, M.D., Raymond S. Greenberg, M.D., and W. Scott Clark, M.S. "Breast Self-Examination and Survival from Breast Cancer." *Cancer* 1988, 62:1389–1396.

3. The Miracle of Mammography

1. Herbert Seidman, M.B.A., Steven Gelb, M.S., Edwin Silverberg, B.S., Nancy LaVerda, M.P.H., and John A. Lubera, B.B.A. "Survival Experience in the Breast Cancer Detection Demonstration Project." *CA* 1987, 37:258–290.
2. Gloria Frankl, M.D. "The Use of Screening Mammography." *Cancer* 1987, 60:1979–1983.

4. Diagnosing the Problem: Breast Biopsy

1. William H. Wolberg, M.D., Martin A. Tanner, Ph.D., and Wei-Yin Loh, Ph.D. "Fine Needle Aspiration for Breast Mass Diagnosis." *Archives of Surgery* 1989, 124:814–818.

5. *Most Lumps* Aren't *Cancer:*
Understanding Fibrocystic Changes

1. J. P. Minton, M.D., M. Foecking, M.D., and D. Webster, M.D., "Responses of Fibrocystic Disease to Caffeine Withdrawal and Correlation of Cyclic Nucleotides with Breast Disease." *American Journal of Obstetrics and Gynecology* 1979, 135:157–158.
2. Flora Lubin, Elaine Ron, Ph.D., Yochanan Wax, Ph.D., Maurice Black, M.D., Michaela Funaro, M.Sc., and Angela Shitrit, M.A. "A Case-Control Study of Caffeine and Methylxanthines in Benign Breast Disease." *Journal of the American Medical Association* 1985, 253:2388–2392.
3. Amos E. Madanes, M.D., and Martin Farber, M.D. "Danazol." *Annals of Internal Medicine* 1982, 96:625–630.

6. *What Is the Risk*
of Getting Breast Cancer?

1. Phyllis A. Wingo, M.S., Peter M. Layde, M.D., Nancy C. Lee, M.D., George L. Rubin, M.B., and Howard W. Ory, M.D. "The Risk of Breast Cancer in Postmenopausal Women Who Have Used Estrogen Replacement Therapy." *Journal of the American Medical Association* 1987, 257:209–215.
2. Leif Bergkvist, M.D., Hans-Olov Adami, M.D., Ingemar Persson, M.D., Robert N. Hoover, M.D., and Catherine Schairer, M.S. "The Risk of Breast Cancer After Estrogen and Estrogen-Progestin Replacement." *New England Journal of Medicine* 1989, 321:293–297.
3. Julie E. Buring, D.Sc., Charles H. Hennekens, M.D., Robert J. Lipnick, D.Sc., Walter Willett, M.D., Meir J. Stampfer, M.D., Bernard A. Rosner, Ph.D., Richard Peto, M.Sc., and Frank E. Speizer, M.D. "A Prospective Cohort Study of Postmenopausal Hormone Use and Risk of

Breast Cancer in U.S. Women." *American Journal of Epidemiology* 1987, 125:939–947.

4. Robert J. Lipnick, D.Sc., Julie E. Buring, D.Sc., Charles H. Hennekens, M.D., Bernard A. Rosner, Ph.D., Walter Willett, M.D., Christopher Bain, M.B., Meir J. Stampfer, M.D., Graham A. Colditz, M.B., Richard Peto, M.Sc., and Frank E. Speizer, M.D. "Oral Contraceptives and Breast Cancer." *Journal of the American Medical Association* 1986, 255:58–61.

5. Richard W. Sattin, M.D., George L. Rubin, M.B., Phyliss A. Wingo, M.D., Linda Webster, M.S.P.H., and Howard W. Ory, M.D. "Oral-Contraceptive Use and the Risk of Breast Cancer." *New England Journal of Medicine* 1986, 315:405–411.

6. Dutzu Rosner, M.D., and Warren W. Lane, Ph.D. "Oral Contraceptive Use Has No Adverse Effect on the Prognosis of Breast Cancer." *Cancer* 1986, 57:591–596.

7. Walter Willett, M.D., Meir J. Stampfer, M.D., G. A. Colditz, M.B., Bernard A. Rosner, Ph.D., Charles H. Hennekens, M.D., and Frank E. Speizer. "Moderate Alcohol Consumption and the Risk of Breast Cancer." *New England Journal of Medicine* 1987, 316:1174–1180.

8. Arthur Schatzkin, M.D., Yvone Jones, Ph.D., Robert N. Hoover, M.D., Philip R. Taylor, M.D., Louise Brinton, Sc.D., Regina G. Ziegler, Ph.D., Elizabeth B. Harvey, Ph.D., Christine L. Carter, Ph.D., Lisa M. Licitra, B.A., Mary C. Dufour, M.D., and David B. Larson, M.D. "Alcohol Consumption and Breast Cancer in the Epidemiologic Follow-up Study of the First National Health and Nutrition Examination Survey." *New England Journal of Medicine* 1987, 316:1169–1173.

9. Randall E. Harris, M.D., and Ernst L. Wynder, M.D. "Breast Cancer and Alcohol Consumption." *Journal of the American Medical Association* 1988, 259:2867–2871.

10. John E. Woods. "Detailed Technique of Subcutaneous Mastectomy

with and without Mastopexy." Annals of Plastic Surgery 1987, 18:51–61.

7. Breast Cancer: After
the Diagnosis

1. Christine L. Carter, Ph.D., Carol Allen, Ph.D., and Donald Henson, M.D. "Relation of Tumor Size, Lymph Node Status, and Survival in 24,740 Breast Cancer Cases." Cancer 1989, 63:181–187.
2. American Joint Committee on Cancer 1989. Staging for Breast Carcinoma. American Cancer Society, Inc. 3rd edition.
3. Bernard Fisher, M.D. "Comparison of Radical Mastectomy with Alternative Treatments for Primary Breast Cancer." Cancer 1977, 39:2827–2839.

8. Basic Information for
the Treatment of Breast Cancer

1. John M. Kurtz, M.D., Robert Amalric, M.D., Gilles Delouche, M.D., Bernard Pierquin, M.D., Jakob Roth, Ph.D., and Jean-Maurice Spitalier, M.D. "The Second Ten Years: Long Term Risks of Breast Conservation and Early Breast Cancer." International Journal of Radiation Oncology 1987, 13:1327–1332.
2. Eleanor D. Montague, M.D., and Gilbert H. Fletcher, M.D. "Local Regional Effectiveness of Surgery and Radiation Therapy in the Treatment of Breast Cancer." Cancer 1985, 55:2266–2272.
3. Avrum Z. Bluming, M.D., et al. "Los Angeles Community Experience. Treatment of Primary Breast Cancer without Mastectomy." Annals of Surgery 1986, 204:136–147.
4. Umberto Veronesi, M.D., Roberto Zucali, M.D., and Marcella Del

Vecchio, Ph.D. "Conservative Treatment of Breast Cancer with the QU.A.R.T Technique." *World Journal of Surgery* 1985, 9:676–681.

5. Bernard Fisher, M.D., "The National Surgical Adjuvant Breast and Bowel Project. Five-Year Results of a Randomized Clinical Trial Comparing Total Mastectomy and Segmental Mastectomy with or without Radiation in the Treatment of Breast Cancer." *New England Journal of Medicine* 1985, 312:665–673.

6. Bernard Fisher, M.D. "The National Surgical Adjuvant Breast and Bowel Project. Ten-Year Results of a Randomized Clinical Trial Comparing Radical Mastectomy and Total Mastectomy with or without Radiation." *New England Journal of Medicine* 1985, 312:674–681.

7. Bernard Fisher, M.D. "The National Surgical Adjuvant Breast and Bowel Project. A Randomized Clinical Trial Evaluating Tamoxifen in the Treatment of Patients with Node-Negative Breast Cancer Who Have Estrogen-Receptor-Positive Tumors." *New England Journal of Medicine* 1989, 320:479–484.

8. Bernard Fisher, M.D. "The National Surgical Adjuvant Breast and Bowel Project. Ten-Year Results from the NSABP Clinical Trial Evaluating the Use of L-Phenylalanine Mustard (L-PAM) in the Management of Primary Breast Cancer." *Journal of Clinical Onology*, 1986, 4:929–941.

9. Bernard Fisher, M.D. "The National Surgical Adjuvant Breast and Bowel Project. A Randomized Clinical Trial Evaluating Sequential Methotrexate and Fluorouracil in the Treatment of Patients with Node-Negative Breast Cancer Who Have Estrogen-Receptor-Negative Tumors." *New England Journal of Medicine* 1989, 320:473–478.

10. The Ludwig Breast Cancer Study Group. "Prolonged Disease-Free Survival After One Course of Perioperative Adjuvant Chemotherapy for Node-Negative Breast Cancer." *New England Journal of Medicine* 1989, 320:491–496.

11. Edward G. Mansour, M.D. "An Intergroup Study. Efficacy of Adjuvant Chemotherapy in High-Risk Node-Negative Breast Cancer." *New England Journal of Medicine* 1989, 320:485–490.

12. *Chemotherapy and You.* U.S. Department of Health and Human Services, N.I.H. Publication No. 86–1136, National Cancer Institute, 1986.

9. Specific Treatment Recommendations for Breast Cancer

1. Philip Nugent, M.D., and Theodore X. O'Connell, M.D. "Breast Cancer and Pregnancy." *Archives of Surgery* 1985, 120:1221–1224.

11. A New Beginning: Breast Reconstruction Surgery

1. R. Barrett Noone, M.D., J. Brein Murphy, M.D., and John W. Little III, M.D. "A 6-Year Experience with the Immediate Reconstruction After Mastectomy for Cancer." *Plastic and Reconstructive Surgery* 1985, 76:258–269.

2. David K. Wellisch, Ph.D., Wendy S. Schain, Ed.D., R. Barrett Noone, M.D., and John W. Little III, M.D. "Psycho-social Correlates of Immediate versus Delayed Reconstruction of the Breast." *Plastic and Reconstructive Surgery* 1985, 76:713–718.

12. Changing the Look of Your Breasts: Enlargement, Reduction, and Breast Lift Surgery

1. Melvin J. Silverstein, M.D., Neal Handel, M.D., Parvis Gamagami, M.D., James R. Waisman, M.D., Eugene D. Gierson, M.D., Robert J.

Rosser, M.D., Robert Steyskal, M.D., and William Colburn, M.D. "Breast Cancer in Women After Augmentation Mammoplasty." *Archives of Surgery* 1988, 123:681–685.

2. *Safety of Silicone Prostheses.* FDA Drug Bulletin, 1989.

Index

Page numbers in *italics* refer to illustrations.